◇ NORMAL VALUES IN PREGNANCY

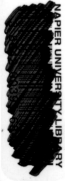
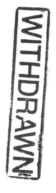

NORMAL VALUES IN PREGNANCY

MM RAMSAY *MA, MD, MRCOG, MRCP*
Fetomaternal Medicine Training Fellow
University Department of Obstetrics and Gynaecology
Queen's Medical Centre
Nottingham, UK

DK JAMES *MA, MD, FRCOG, DCH*
Professor of Fetomaternal Medicine
University Department of Obstetrics and Gynaecology
Queen's Medical Centre
Nottingham, UK

CP WEINER *MD*
Professor and Chairman, Department of Obstetrics,
Gynecology and Reproductive Sciences
University of Maryland School of Medicine
Baltimore, Maryland, USA

PJ STEER *BSc, MD, FRCOG*
Professor, Academic Department of Obstetrics and
Gynaecology
Charing Cross and Westminster Medical School
Chelsea and Westminster Hospital, London, UK

B GONIK *MD*
Professor and Vice Chairman
Department of Obstetrics and Gynecology
Wayne State University School of Medicine
Grace Hospital, Detroit, Michigan, USA

WB Saunders Company Limited ◆ London · Philadelphia · Toronto · Sydney · Tokyo

W.B Saunders Company Ltd 24–28 Oval Road
London NW1 7DX, UK

The Curtis Center
Independence Square West
Philadelphia, PA 19106–3399,
USA

Harcourt Brace & Company
55 Horner Avenue
Toronto, Ontario M8Z 4X6,
Canada

Harcourt Brace & Company, Australia
30–52 Smidmore Street
Marrickville, NSW 2204,
Australia

Harcourt Brace & Company, Japan
Ichibancho Central Building,
22–1 Ichibancho
Chiyoda-ku, Tokyo 102, Japan

British Library Cataloguing in Publication Data is available.

ISBN 0-7020-2021-4

This book is printed on acid-free paper

Typeset by Phoenix Photosetting, Chatham, Kent
Printed in Great Britain by WBC Book Manufacturers Ltd, Bridgend, Mid Glamorgan

CONTENTS

INTRODUCTION

Pregnancy results in profound changes in maternal physiology and metabolism. Without knowledge of these changes and the different normal values which are appropriate in pregnancy and which may vary with gestational age, it is impossible to diagnose accurately and manage maternal and fetal disorders.

The fetus is now accessible via ultrasound and ultrasound-guided invasive procedures and can be subjected to detailed evaluation. Detailed knowledge of fetal morphology, physiology and growth is now considered essential for an acceptable standard of care.

For these reasons, *Normal Values in Pregnancy* should be immediately at hand for all professionals involved in pregnancy care – in the clinic, ward and home. The book started life as an appendix (compiled by Margaret Ramsay) to our postgraduate textbook, *High Risk Pregnancy – Management Options*, but it was greeted with such acclaim that we thought it important to produce this updated and easily portable version. We have included new data, converted data previously published as tables into user-friendly graphs, and have supplied, where possible, alternative units of measurement.

At present, data on many normal ranges are deficient or limited and occasionally unreliable. We have sought to draw the reader's attention to these issues in the comments for each section. However, we can only rely on studies performed and published to date. Much basic work remains to be done and we hope to incorporate this in future editions. Thus, we would welcome correspondence from readers with such data. Such contributions would be fully acknowledged.

The definition of 'normal' is contentious. It can mean 'lack of pathology'. It can mean the 'best performer' or 'ideal measure'. Alternatively, it can be defined statistically within certain limits (e.g. 10th/90th or 5th/95th or 3rd/97th centiles or within 2 standard deviations of the mean). In this text, we have had to report the values as they appear in the literature, which means that we have been unable to be consistent in the way the ranges are expressed. Furthermore, these ranges do not always reflect the levels at which pathology occurs. We hope to standardize the information in later editions as better information becomes available.

In summary, we believe we have produced a unique, comprehensive and practical publication covering a dynamic area.

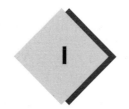

MATERNAL VALUES

PHYSIOLOGY

Nutrition

Weight gain

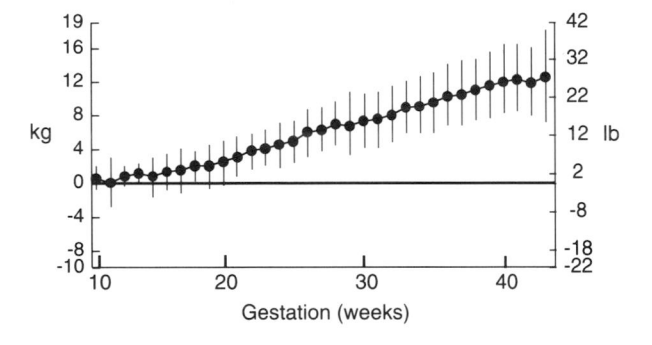

Figure 1. Maternal weight gain (mean ± SD) in 988 normal women who had uneventful pregnancies; all booked at < 20 weeks and delivered between 37 and 41 weeks. (Longitudinal study.) *Data source:* ref. 1, with permission.

	Recommended total weight gain	
Weight-for-height category	kg	lb
Low (BMI <19.8)	12.5–18	28–40
Normal (BMI 19.8–26.0)	11.5–16	25–35
High (BMI 26.0–29.0)	7–11.5	15–25
Obese (BMI >29.0)	7	15

BMI=(weight/height^2)

Figure 2. Recommended total body weight gain ranges for women during pregnancy with a singleton gestation, classified by pre-pregnancy body mass index (BMI). *Data source:* ref. 2, with permission.

Comment: Average total weight gain during pregnancy is approximately 10 kg. Low weight gain during pregnancy in non-obese women has been associated with delivery of small-for-gestational-age infants[3]. However, overweight women often deliver large-for-gestational-age infants, regardless of their weight gain during pregnancy[3].

Nutritional requirements

Nutrient (unit)	Pregnant	Lactating
Energy (kcal)	+300	+500
Protein (g)	60	65
Fat-soluble vitamins		
Vitamin A (µg retinol equivalents)	800	1300
Vitamin D (µg as cholecalciferol)	10	10
Vitamin E (mg α-tocopherol equivalents)	10	12
Vitamin K (µg)	65	65
Water-soluble vitamins		
Vitamin C (mg)	70	95
Thiamin (mg)	1.5	1.6
Riboflavin (mg)	1.6	1.8
Niacin (mg niacin equivalent)	17	20
Vitamin B_6 (mg)	2.2	2.1
Folate (µg)	400	280
Vitamin B_{12} (µg)	2.2	2.6
Minerals		
Calcium (mg)	1200	1200
Phosphorus (mg)	1200	1200
Magnesium (mg)	300	355
Iron (mg)	30	15
Zinc (mg)	15	19
Iodine (µg)	175	200
Selenium (µg)	65	75

Figure 3. Recommended daily dietary allowances and energy intakes for women whilst pregnant and lactating. These should be used as a guide to nutritional requirements when formulating a balanced diet. *Data source:* ref. 4, with permission.

Comment: The increased requirements during pregnancy for vitamins and minerals can usually be met from the diet, thus routine supplementation with multivitamin preparations is not necessary. However, periconceptual supplementation with folic acid for all women in pregnancy is now advocated in an attempt to reduce the incidence of neural tube defects. Vitamin supplementation should be considered in women with inadequate standard diets, heavy smokers, drug or alcohol-abusers, or those with multiple pregnancies. Excessive intake (i.e. more than twice the recommended daily allowance) of vitamins (fat or water-soluble) may have toxic effects.

Cardiovascular Function

Blood pressure

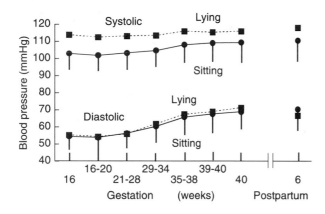

Figure 4. Blood pressure measurements (mean and SD) from a longitudinal study of 226 primigravidae whose first attendance at the antenatal clinic was before 20 weeks of pregnancy. Their mean age was 24.3 (SD 4.9) years. Blood pressure measurements were taken with the London School of Hygiene sphygmomano-meter to avoid terminal digit preference and observer bias; diastolic pressures were recorded at the point of muffling (phase 4). *Data source*: ref. 5, with permission.

Comment: Systolic pressure changes little during pregnancy, but diastolic pressure falls markedly towards mid-pregnancy, then rising to near non-pregnant levels by term. Thus there is a widening of the pulse pressure for most of the pregnancy.

Cardiovascular Function

Pulse rate

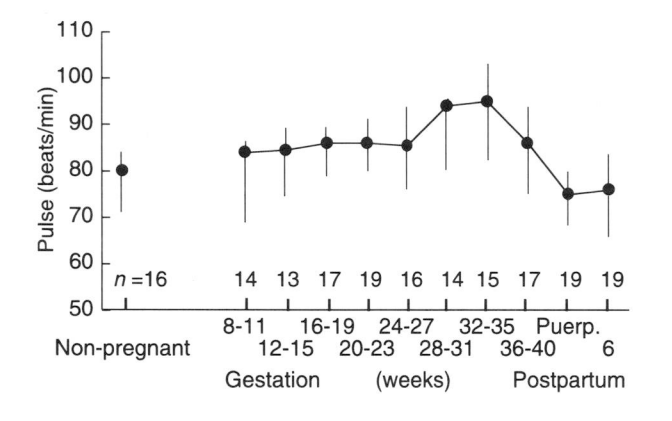

Figure 5. Pulse rate (median and IQ ranges) from a longitudinal study of 20 healthy women recruited in early pregnancy and studied every 2 weeks thereafter; 'non-pregnant' measurements were made 8–12 months after delivery. All women finished the study but not all participated in every visit. *Data source*: ref. 6, with permission.

Comment: The typical increase in heart rate during pregnancy is approximately 15 beats/min, present from as early as 4 weeks after the last menstrual period[7].

Cardiac output

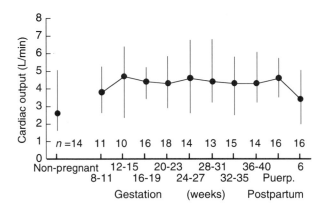

Figure 6. Cardiac output (median and IQ ranges) from a longitudinal study of 20 healthy women recruited in early pregnancy and studied every 2 weeks thereafter; 'non-pregnant' measurements were made 8–12 months after delivery. All women finished the study but not all participated in every visit. Cardiac output was measured by an indirect Fick method. *Data source*: ref. 6, with permission.

Comment: Cardiac output increases significantly during the first trimester and thereafter remains elevated until the puerperium. When changes in body weight are taken into consideration, it is apparent that cardiac output reaches maximal values between 12 and 15 weeks and thereafter declines gradually towards term.

Cardiovascular Function

Invasive monitoring

	Non-pregnant	Pregnant
Cardiac output (L/min)	4.3 ± 0.9	6.2 ± 1.0
Heart rate (beats/min)	71 ± 10	83 ± 10
Systemic vascular resistance (dyne cm s^{-5})	1530 ± 520	1210 ± 266
Pulmonary vascular resistance (dyne cm s^{-5})	119 ± 47	78 ± 22
Colloid oncotic pressure (mmHg)	20.8 ± 1.0	18.0 ± 1.5
Colloid oncotic pressure– pulmonary capillary wedge pressure (mmHg)	14.5 ± 2.5	10.5 ± 2.7
Mean arterial pressure (mmHg)	86.4 ± 7.5	90.3 ± 5.8
Pulmonary capillary wedge pressure (mmHg)	6.3 ± 2.1	7.5 ± 1.8
Central venous pressure (mmHg)	3.7 ± 2.6	3.6 ± 2.5
Left ventricular stroke work index (g m m^{-2})	41 ± 8	48 ± 6

Figure 7. Study involving 10 healthy, primigravid women with a singleton pregnancy examined between 36 and 38 weeks gestation and then again between 11 and 13 weeks postpartum. All women were less than 26 years old, non-smokers, not anemic and there was normal fetal anatomy, growth and amniotic fluid volume. A pulmonary artery catheter was placed via the sub-clavian vein and baseline hemodynamic assessment was made in the left lateral position after 30 minutes rest. Cardiac output was measured with a thermo-dilution technique (and for each subject the result represented the mean of five independent measurements with the highest and lowest values excluded); central pressures were measured over three consecutive respiratory cycles. Results quoted are mean ± SD. *Data source:* ref. 8, with permission.

Comment: Systemic vascular resistance is 21% lower and pulmonary resistance is 34% lower in late third trimester than in the non-pregnant state. Both colloid oncotic pressure and the colloid oncotic–pulmonary capillary wedge pressure gradient are also lower (by 14% and 28% respectively). There are no significant changes in the third trimester with respect to mean arterial pressure, central venous pressure, pulmonary capillary wedge pressure or left ventricular stroke work index. These results indicate that both systemic and pulmonary vascular beds accomodate higher vascular volumes at normal pressures during pregnancy, the ventricles are dilated and cardiac contractility does not change significantly. Since the colloid oncotic pressure–pulmonary capillary wedge pressure gradient is reduced in pregnancy, any increase in cardiac pre-load or any alteration in pulmonary capillary permeability will predispose to pulmonary edema.

Pulmonary Function and Respiration
Arterial blood gases

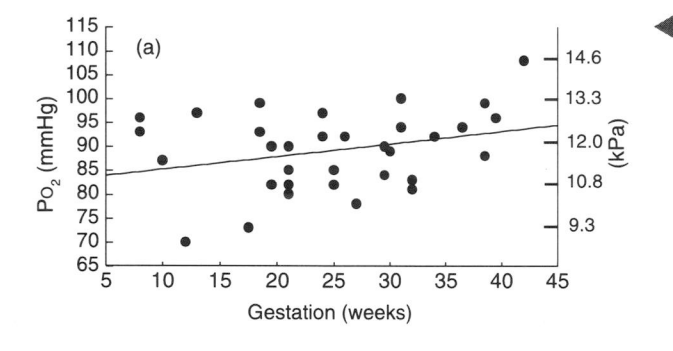

Figure 8. Arterial blood gas pressures – (a) oxygen (PO_2), (b) carbon dioxide (PCO_2) and (c) standard bicarbonate (individual values, with regression lines shown) from a cross-sectional study of 37 women between 8 and 42 weeks of pregnancy. Blood sampling was done from a cannula inserted into the brachial artery under local anesthesia, after 30 minutes rest in a quiet, darkened room. *Data source*: ref. 9, with permission of Elsevier Science NL, Amsterdam, The Netherlands.

Comment: Arterial pH was found to be constant (7.47) during pregnancy in this study. PCO_2 and standard bicarbonate showed significant decrease with advancing gestation, but PO_2 levels did not alter significantly.

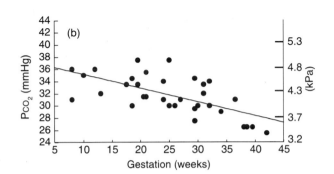

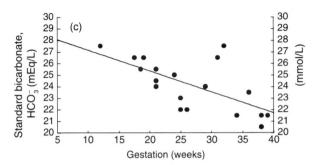

Pulmonary Function and Respiration

Transcutaneous gases

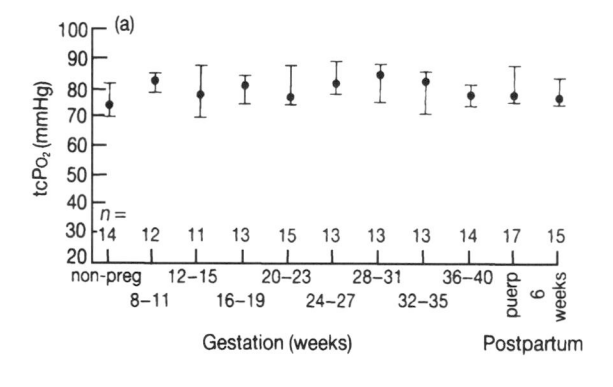

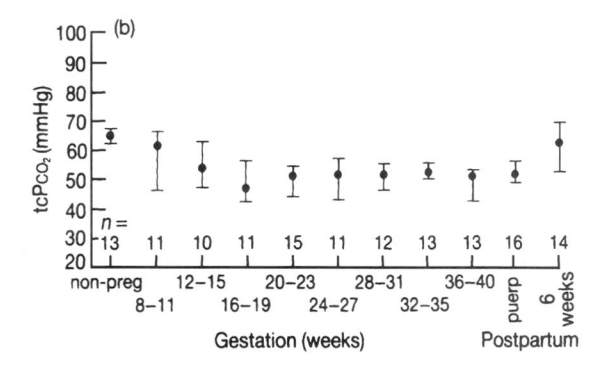

Figure 9. (a) Transcutaneous oxygen (tcPo₂) and (b) carbon dioxide (tcPco₂) pressures (median and IQ ranges) from a longitudinal study of 20 healthy women recruited in early pregnancy and studied every 2 weeks thereafter; 'non-pregnant' measurements were made 8–12 months after delivery. All women finished the study but not all participated in every visit. *Data source*: ref. 6, with permission.

Comment: Transcutaneous Pco₂ is higher than arterial Pco₂ due to temperature differences between the skin surface and blood, as well as addition of CO₂ by skin metabolism (conversion factor *approx* 1.4)[6]. Transcutaneous Po₂ values in adults are 10–20% lower than arterial Po₂ values. In this study the rise in tcPo₂ and fall in tcPco₂ during pregnancy were both significant.

Respiration rate

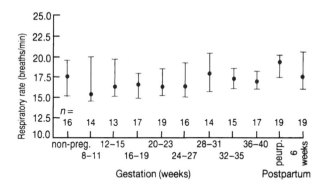

Figure 10. Respiration rate (median and IQ ranges) from a longitudinal study of 20 healthy women recruited in early pregnancy and studied every 2 weeks thereafter; 'non-pregnant' measurements were made 8–12 months after delivery. All women finished the study but not all participated in every visit. *Data source*: ref. 6, with permission.

Comment: Respiration rate is similar in pregnant and non-pregnant women.

Pulmonary Function and Respiration

Tidal volume

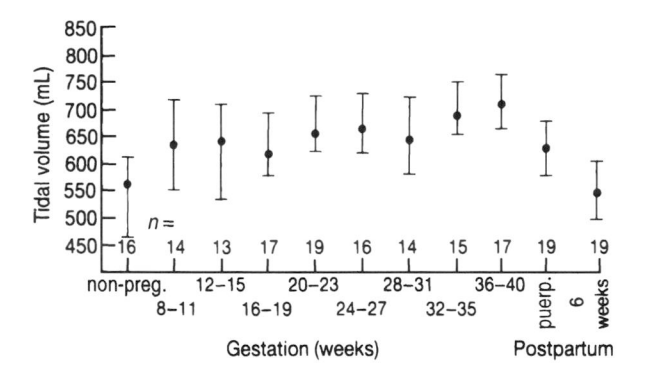

Figure 11. Tidal volume (medium and IQ ranges) from a longitudinal study of 20 healthy women recruited in early pregnancy and studied every 2 weeks thereafter; 'non-pregnant' measurements were made 8–12 months after delivery. All women finished the study but not all participated in every visit. *Data source*: ref. 6, with permission.

Comment: Tidal volume increases early in pregnancy and continues to rise until term; overall, there is a 30–40% rise. By 6–8 weeks postpartum, tidal volumes have returned to non-pregnant values. Minute ventilation rises in parallel with tidal volume; typical values are 7.5 L/min for a non-pregnant woman, and 10.5 L/min in late pregnancy[10].

	During pregnancy			After delivery
	10 weeks	24 weeks	36 weeks	10 weeks postpartum
Vital capacity (L)	3.8	3.9	4.1	3.8
Inspiratory capacity (L)	2.6	2.7	2.9	2.5
Expiratory reserve volume (L)	1.2	1.2	1.2	1.3
Residual volume (L)	1.2	1.1	1.0	1.2

Figure 12. Respiratory volumes (mean values) from a longitudinal study of eight healthy women, aged 18–29 years, studied through pregnancy and then again 10 weeks postpartum. All tests were done in the sitting position. *Data source*: ref. 10, with permission.

Comment: Some women increase their vital capacity (by 100–200 mL) during pregnancy, but the converse has been demonstrated in obese women[11]. Anatomical changes (flaring of the lower ribs, a rise in the diaphragm and increase in transverse diameter of the chest) are responsible for the alterations in lung volume subdivisions[11]. Forced expiratory volume in one second (FEV_1) and peak expiratory flow rate (PFR) are unaffected by normal pregnancy[10]. Gas transfer factor (i.e. pulmonary diffusing capacity with carbon monoxide) decreases in pregnancy[10]. This has been attributed to altered mucopolysaccharides in the alveolar capillary walls, as well as a lower circulating hemoglobin.

Chromosomal Abnormalities

Chromosomal Abnormalities

Figure 13. Risk of having a pregnancy associated with Down's syndrome according to maternal age at time of birth. *Data source*: ref. 12, with permission.

Maternal age at delivery (years)	Risk of Down's syndrome
15	1: 1578
20	1: 1528
25	1: 1351
30	1: 909
31	1: 796
32	1: 683
33	1: 574
34	1: 474
35	1: 384
36	1: 307
37	1: 242
38	1: 189
39	1: 146
40	1: 112
41	1: 85
42	1: 65
43	1: 49
44	1: 37
45	1: 28
46	1: 21
47	1: 15
48	1: 11
49	1: 8
50	1: 6

Maternal age	Rate per 1000				
	Trisomy 21	Trisomy 18	Trisomy 13	XXY	All chromosome anomalies
35	3.9	0.5	0.2	0.5	8.7
36	5.0	0.7	0.3	0.6	10.1
37	6.4	1.0	0.4	0.8	12.2
38	8.1	1.4	0.5	1.1	14.8
39	10.4	2.0	0.8	1.4	18.4
40	13.3	2.8	1.1	1.8	23.0
41	16.9	3.9	1.5	2.4	29.0
42	21.6	5.5	2.1	3.1	37.0
43	27.4	7.6		4.1	45.0
44	34.8			5.4	50.0
45	44.2			7.0	62.0
46	55.9			9.1	77.0
47	70.4			11.9	96.0

Figure 14. Chromosomal abnormalities by maternal age at time of amniocentesis at 16 weeks gestation (expressed as rate per 1000). *Data source*: ref. 13, with permission.

Comment: The incidence of chromosomal disorders rises with increasing maternal age, but is not influenced by paternal age[13]. Trisomy 21 (Down's syndrome) is the most important numerically of these disorders, with an overall population incidence of 1 in 650 live births. Trisomies 13, 18 and 22 are rare as live births. Other autosomal trisomies are non-viable and are commonly found in spontaneous abortions.

Chromosomal Abnormalities

BIOCHEMISTRY

Hepatic Function

Total serum protein and albumin

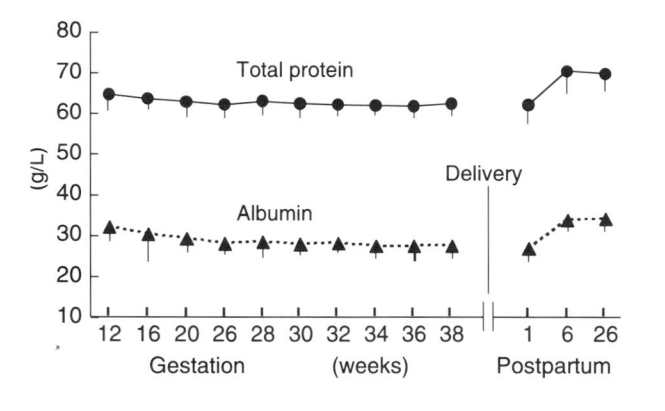

Figure 15. Total serum protein and albumin (mean and SD) from a longitudinal study of 83 healthy pregnant women (77 of whom were primigravidae), recruited at 12 weeks gestation. Samples were collected every 4 weeks during pregnancy, 7 days postpartum, then at 6 and 26 weeks postpartum. *Data source*: ref. 14, with permission.

Comment: Decreased total serum protein and albumin concentrations in pregnancy are associated with a decrease in colloid osmotic pressure[14]. Serum immunoglobulin levels do not change significantly in pregnancy[15].

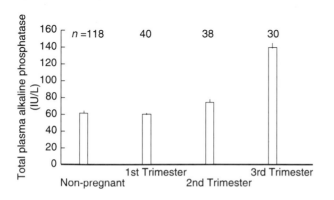

Figure 16. Total alkaline phosphatase (mean and SEM) from a cross-sectional study of 108 normal women attending a hospital antenatal clinic in Nigeria; the non-pregnant controls of similar age were patients attending the gynecological clinic. No patients were clinically anemic and all were normotensive. *Data source*: ref. 16, with permission.

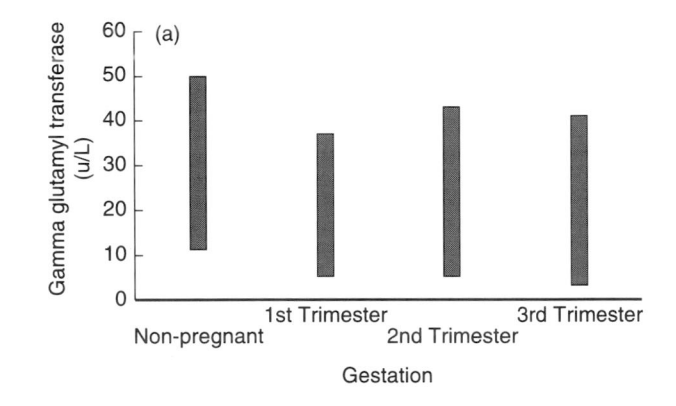

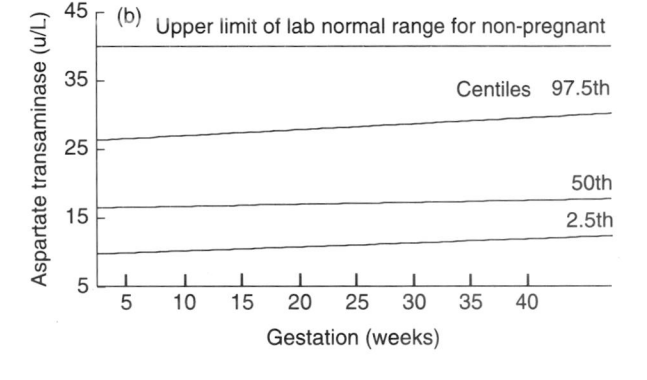

▲

Figure 17. (a) Serum gamma glutamyl transferase (GGT), (b) aspartate transaminase (AST), (c) alanine transaminase (ALT) and (d) bilirubin (95% reference ranges) from a cross-sectional study of 430 women with uncomplicated singleton pregnancy. All subjects were free from hypertension or liver disease and none was taking drugs associated with liver dysfunction or consuming more than 10 units of alcohol per week. Data for GGT were not normally distributed and the results presented are calculated from the non-parametric determination of percentiles. Data for AST, ALT and bilirubin were normally distributed after logarithmic transformation, allowing gestation-specific centiles to be calculated. *Data source*: ref. 17, with permission.

▼

Comment: Total plasma alkaline phosphatase (AP) levels are approximately doubled by late pregnancy. Almost half of the total plasma AP in pregnancy is placental AP isoenzyme, but bone AP isoenzyme levels are also markedly increased; liver AP isoenzyme levels do not change significantly in pregnancy[16]. Serum gamma glutamyl transferase (GGT) and transaminase levels overall are lower in pregnancy than in the non-pregnant adult population. There are not significant gestational changes in GGT, AST or ALT, nor during labor or the puerperium[18]. Bilirubin levels remain within normal adult levels during pregnancy[19]. No data are available regarding serum amylase in pregnancy, but decreased concentration may be expected as a dilutional effect. There are considerable differences between laboratories with regard to liver enzyme assays and hence 'normal ranges' in the adult population; these should be borne in mind when interpreting individual results from pregnant women.

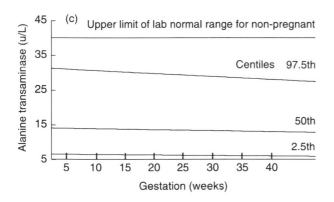

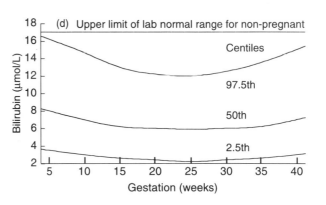

Hepatic Function

Lipids: cholesterol and triglyceride

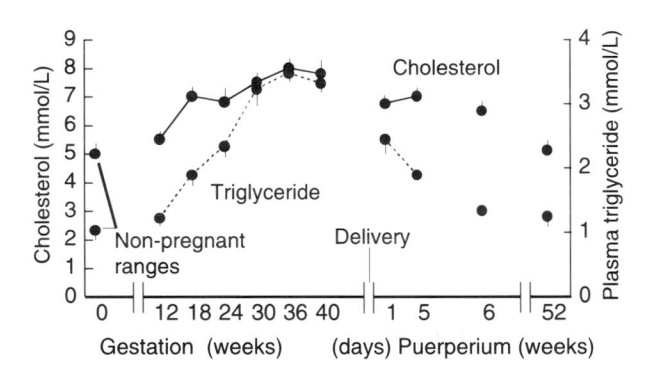

Figure 18. Plasma cholesterol and triglyceride levels (mean and SEM) from a longitudinal study of 43 women aged 20–41 years. Samples were taken following an overnight fast and 10 minutes supine rest at 4–6 weekly intervals through pregnancy, during labor and the puerperium; also 12 months after delivery in 14 of the subjects. The non-pregnant reference samples were from 15 subjects of comparable age. No dietary restrictions were imposed. *Data source*: ref. 20, with permission.

Comment: Plasma cholesterol doubles and there is a three-fold increase in plasma triglyceride concentration during pregnancy. The lipid content of the low density lipoproteins increases in pregnancy, as does high density lipoprotein triglyceride content[20]. Serum lipid levels fall rapidly after delivery, but both cholesterol and triglyceride concentrations remain elevated at 6–7 weeks postpartum. Lactation does not influence lipid levels[20].

Serum urate

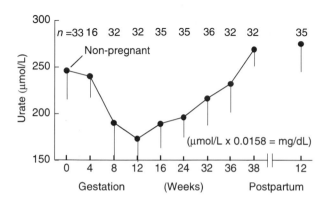

Non-pregnant

$(\mu mol/L \times 0.0158 = mg/dL)$

Gestation (Weeks) Postpartum

Figure 19. Serum urate (mean and SD) from a longitudinal study of 31 healthy women, aged 23–37 years, five of whom were studied during two pregnancies. They were studied pre-conceptually, at least 3 months after stopping oral contraceptives (if used), in the luteal phase of their menstrual cycle, then monthly during pregnancy and again 12 weeks postpartum. All samples were taken between 0900 and 0930 h, after overnight fasting. *Data source*: ref. 21, with permission.

Comment: Serum urate levels decrease during the first trimester, probably due to altered renal handling of uric acid[21]. During late pregnancy, serum urate rises to reach levels higher than non-pregnant values at term; these may remain elevated for 12 weeks after delivery[21].

Serum osmolality, electrolytes and urea

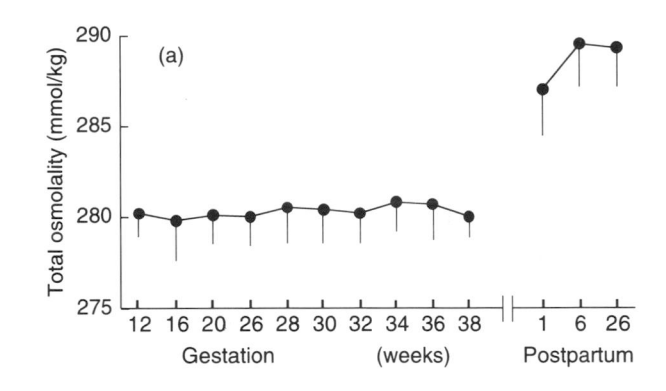 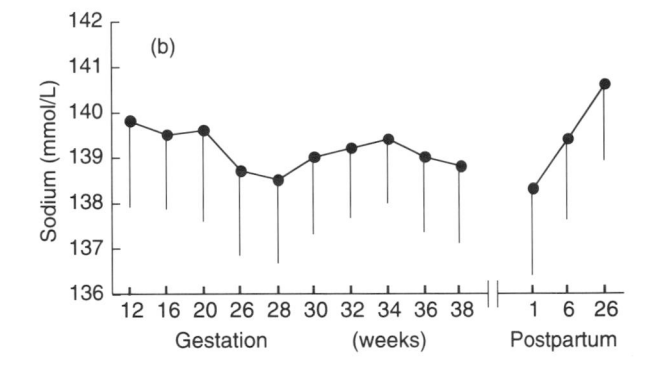

Figure 20. Serum (a) osmolality, (b–d) electrolytes and (e) urea (mean and SD) from a longitudinal study of 83 healthy pregnant women (77 of whom were primigravidae), recruited at 12 weeks gestation. Samples were collected every 4 weeks during pregnancy, 7 days postpartum, then at 6 and 26 weeks postpartum. *Data source*: ref. 14, with permission.

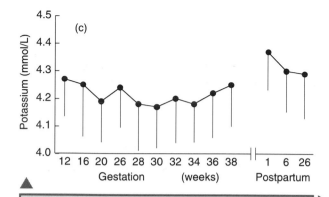

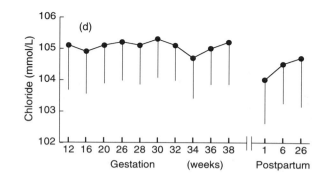

Comment: Total osmolality falls by the end of the first trimester to a nadir 8–10 mmol/kg below non-pregnant values. The major serum electrolytes (sodium, potassium, chloride) have almost unchanged concentrations during pregnancy. Bicarbonate and phosphate concentrations decline during pregnancy[22]. Both plasma urea and creatinine fall during pregnancy; typical mean (SD) values for plasma creatinine are 60 (8), 54 (10) and 64 (9) µmol/L in first, second and third trimesters respectively, rising to 73 (10) µmol/L by 6 weeks postpartum[23,24]; (see also Figure 21b).

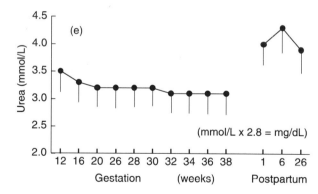

Renal Function

BIOCHEMISTRY

Creatinine clearance and serum creatinine

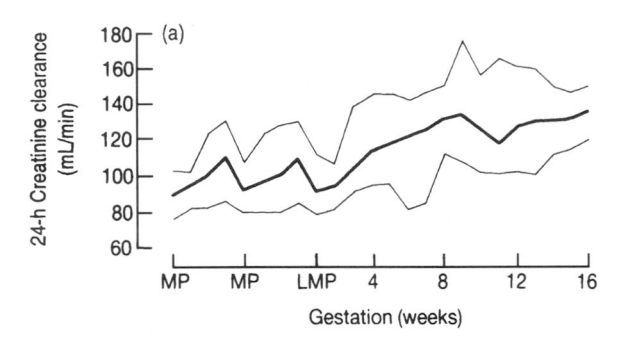

Figure 21. (a) Creatinine clearance (mean and range) in early pregnancy from a longitudinal study of nine healthy women, recruited prior to pregnancy. Measurements of 24-h creatinine clearance were made weekly, through the different phases of the menstrual cycle and up to 16 weeks gestation. No diet, fluid or exercise restrictions were imposed. *Data source*: ref. 25, with permission. (b) Creatinine clearance and serum creatinine (mean ± SEM) in the second and third trimesters from a longitudinal study of 10 healthy pregnant women. Creatinine clearance measurements were made once between 25 and 28 weeks gestation, then weekly from 32 weeks until delivery and finally once between 8 and 12 weeks postpartum. *Data source*: ref. 26, with permission.

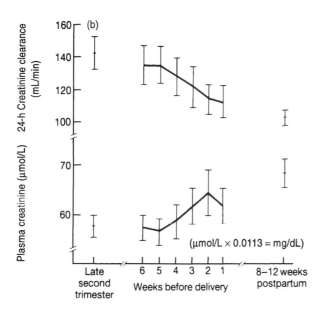

Comment: Glomerular filtration rate (GFR) and effective renal plasma flow increase in early pregnancy to levels approximately 50% above non-pregnant values; in the third trimester, GFR declines by about 15%[26]. 24-h creatinine clearance measurements mirror these changes. During the menstrual cycle, there is a 20% mean increase in creatinine clearance between the week of menstruation and the late luteal phase[25].

Urine composition: glucose, amino acids and protein

Comment: Glycosuria is common in pregnancy in individuals whose plasma glucose concentrations and glucose tolerance tests are normal. It is thought to arise because of increased glomerular filtration plus decreased tubular resorption of glucose[27]. Aminoaciduria has also been demonstrated during pregnancy[28] and there is an increase in urinary albumin excretion[29].

Carbohydrate Metabolism

Fasting plasma glucose

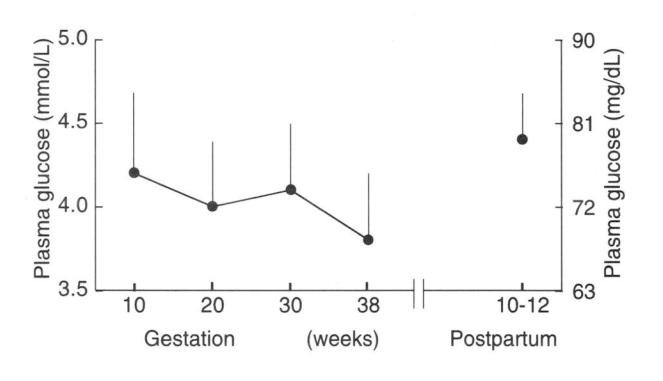

Figure 22. Longitudinal study of plasma glucose levels (mean and SD) following an overnight fast (of at least 10 hours duration) in 19 healthy women, none of whom was obese or had a family history of diabetes mellitus. *Data source*: ref. 30, with permission.

Comment: Plasma glucose levels fall with advancing gestation. In most women, the fall has taken place by the end of the first trimester[30]. Plasma insulin levels rise in the third trimester[30].

Glucose tolerance test (GTT)

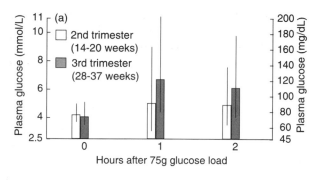

(a)

2nd trimester (14-20 weeks)

3rd trimester (28-37 weeks)

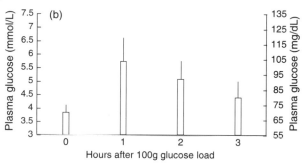

(b)

Figure 23. (a) Plasma glucose values (median, 2.5 and 97.5 centiles) after a 75 g oral glucose load. Cross-sectional study of 111 healthy women under the age of 35 years, weighing less than 85.0 kg, with singleton pregnancies (n=43 and 168 in second and third trimesters respectively). None had a personal or family history of diabetes mellitus. *Data source*: ref. 31, with permission. (b) Plasma glucose values (mean and SD) after a 100 g oral glucose load. Study involving 752 unselected pregnancies (n=20, 339 and 393 in the first, second and third trimesters respectively). *Data source*: ref. 32, with permission.

Comment: Women in the third trimester have decreased glucose tolerance, as judged by criteria used to diagnose diabetes outside pregnancy. It has been proposed that gestational diabetes may be diagnosed when two or more of the following plasma glucose levels are found in a 100 g GTT: ≥ 105 mg/dL (fasting), ≥ 190 mg/dL (1 h), 165 mg/dL (2 h), ≥ 145 mg/dL (3 h). These values are 5.8 mmol/L (fasting), 10.6 mmol/L (1 h), 9.2 mmol/L (2 h), 8.1 mmol/L (3 h)[131].

Serum fructosamine, glycosylated hemoglobin

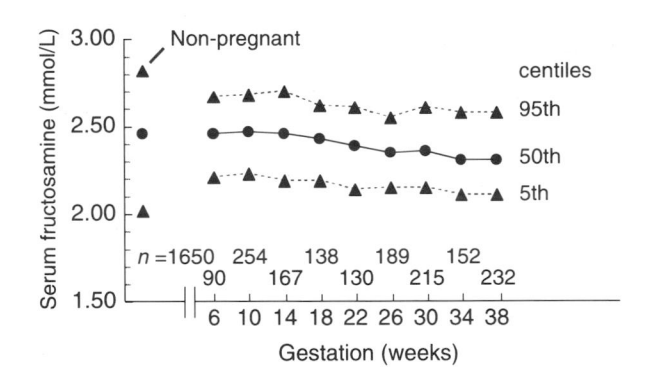

Figure 24. Serum fructosamine (median, 5th and 95th centiles) from a cross-sectional study of 1200 pregnant women at different gestational ages, compared with 1650 non-pregnant women, aged between 15 and 40 years. Women with known diabetes or previous gestational diabetes were excluded from the study. *Data source*: ref. 33, with permission.

Comment: Serum fructosamine concentrations are significantly lower in the second and third trimester than in the first trimester or non-pregnant state. Falling total protein and albumin concentrations in pregnancy may contribute to this reduction in serum fructosamine levels[33]. Values for glycosylated hemoglobin (Hb A_1 and Hb A_{1c}) during pregnancy in healthy women have been shown in some studies to be lower in the first and second trimesters[34] but in other studies to be similar to values found in non-pregnant women[35].

HEMATOLOGY

White Cell Count (total and differential)

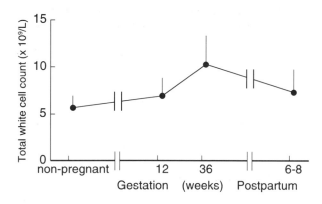

Figure 25. Total white cell count (mean and SD) from a longitudinal study of 24 women recruited at 12 weeks, who delivered after 37 weeks. 'Non-pregnant' samples were taken 4–6 months post-delivery. Samples were analyzed in a Coulter Counter. *Data source*: ref. 36, with permission.

Comment: Supplementation with iron and folate does not affect total white cell count (WBC) during or after pregnancy. Pregnancy-related changes in WBC are still present 6–8 weeks post-delivery. Another (cross-sectional) study found no change in numbers of circulating lymphocytes and monocytes, but decreased eosinophils in the third trimester[37]. Immature granulocytes (myelocytes and metamyelocytes) are found frequently in peripheral blood smears during pregnancy [37,38]. There are no specific data regarding WBC during labor and the early puerperium; however, transiently high values (even up to 25 x 10^9/L) are commonly found.

Hemoglobin and Red Blood Cell Indices

(a)

Parameter	Non-pregnant (SD)	12 weeks (SD)	36 weeks (SD)	Postpartum (SD)
Red blood cell count (x 10^{12}/L)	4.688 (0.309)	4.008 (0.247)	3.880 (0.304)	4.493 (0.338)
Hemoglobin concentration (g/dL)	13.30 (0.77)	12.03 (0.70)	11.07 (0.84)	12.69 (0.92)
Hematocrit (L/L)	0.3936 (0.0233)	0.3515 (0.0226)	0.3311 (0.0232)	0.3787 (0.0289)
Mean cell volume (fL)	83.7 (3.1)	86.2 (3.6)	85.0 (5.3)	84.1 (3.8)
Mean cell hemoglobin (pg)	28.39 (1.06)	30.07 (1.16)	28.65 (2.00)	28.23 (1.45)
Mean cell hemoglobin concentration (g/dL)	33.75 (0.68)	34.23 (1.13)	33.46 (0.82)	33.47 (0.93)

◀ **Figure 26.** (a) Hemoglobin and red cell indices (mean and SD) from a longitudinal study of women recruited at 12 weeks who delivered after 37 weeks (n=24). **No iron or folate supplements were given.** 'Non-pregnant' samples were taken 4–6 months post-delivery. Samples were analyzed in a Coulter Counter. (b) Hemoglobin and red cell indices (mean and SD) from a longitudinal study of women recruited at 12 weeks who delivered after 37 weeks (n=21). **All were given iron and folate supplements** from 12 weeks gestation. 'Non-pregnant' samples were taken 4–6 months post-delivery. Samples were analyzed in a Coulter Counter. *Data source*: ref. 36, with permission.

(b)

Parameter	Non-pregnant (SD)	12 weeks (SD)	36 weeks (SD)	Postpartum (SD)
Red blood cell count (x 10^{12}/L)	4.621 (0.238)	4.109 (0.227)	4.119 (0.246)	4.370 (0.169)
Hemoglobin concentration (g/dL)	13.42 (0.66)	12.06 (0.57)	12.66 (0.81)	13.03 (0.45)
Hematocrit (L/L)	0.3971 (0.0190)	0.3539 (0.020)	0.3666 (0.020)	0.3880 (0.0123)
Mean cell volume (fL)	85.7 (2.2)	86.0 (3.3)	88.8 (2.9)	88.4 (3.3)
Mean cell hemoglobin (pg)	29.00 (0.77)	29.43 (1.03)	30.76 (1.24)	29.86 (1.20)
Mean cell hemoglobin concentration (g/dL)	33.63 (0.69)	34.05 (1.08)	34.50 (0.82)	33.59 (0.66)

Comment: Hemoglobin concentration falls in the first trimester, whether or not iron and folate supplements are given. Pregnancy-induced hematological changes are still present 6–8 weeks postpartum.

Platelet Count and Indices

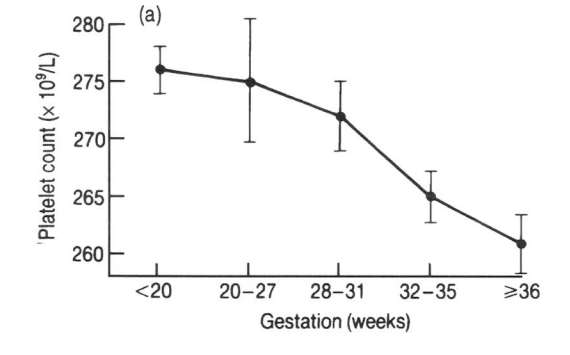

Figure 27. (a) Platelet count and (b) mean platelet volume (mean ± SEM) during pregnancy. Study was largely cross-sectional in design (2881 samples from 2114 women). Samples were analyzed in a Coulter Counter. At the end of the study, any patients who had developed hypertension were excluded. *Data source*: ref. 39, with permission.

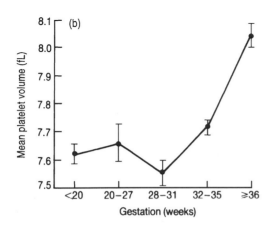

Comment: It has been suggested that there is hyper-destruction of platelets in pregnancy, with a consequent decrease in platelet lifespan. Young platelets are known to be larger than old platelets. Another study[40] of longitudinal design, but with much smaller numbers (*n*=44) did not find evidence of significant change in the platelet count with gestational age.

Iron Metabolism

(a)

Patients	Hb (g/dL)	Serum iron (µmol/L)	Transferrin/ TIBC saturation (%)	Serum ferritin (µg/L)
Not treated (*n*=30)				
First trimester	12.9	23	36	96
Term	12.0	14	13	13
Given FeSO₄ (*n*=82)				
First trimester	12.5	22	33	67
Term	12.5	25	27	41

Figure 28. Mean hemoglobin (Hb) and iron indices from a longitudinal study of women recruited in the first trimester. At the start, 72 were randomized to the 'no treatment' group, but any whose Hb fell below 11 g/dL were prescribed ferrous sulfate 60 mg t.d.s.; thus only 30 progressed through pregnancy without iron supplements. In all subjects studied, serum ferritin rose rapidly postpartum, reaching similar values to those found in early pregnancy by 5–8 weeks after delivery (NB. no iron supplements were given following delivery). *Data source*: ref. 41, with permission.

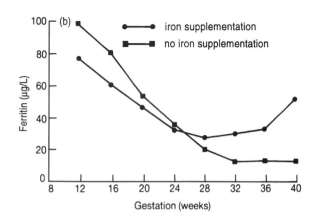

Comment: Iron stores (as indicated by serum ferritin) become depleted during pregnancy, whether or not iron supplements are given.

Serum and Red Cell Folate

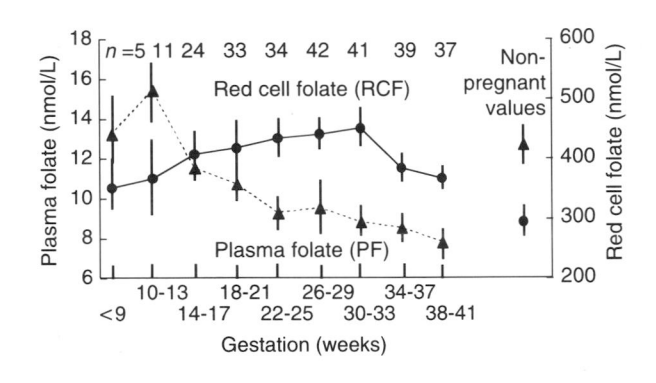

Figure 29. Longitudinal study of plasma and red cell folate levels (mean ± SEM) during singleton pregnancy; all women were taking iron supplements from approximately 12 weeks gestation, but none took folate supplements (*n*=43). Samples were taken after overnight fasting, with patients seated. Non-pregnant reference samples were from 50 healthy women (non-lactating) aged 19–37 years, taken 3–5 hours following their last meal. None of the women developed anemia during pregnancy (Hemoglobin and mean cell volume remained stable). *Data source*: ref. 42, with permission.

Comment: In other studies, red cell folate has been shown to have a slight downward trend with advancing gestation and those patients with low red cell folate at the beginning of pregnancy develop megaloblastic anemia in the third trimester[43]. These differences may relate to dietary folate intake. Plasma and red cell folate values are similar in pregnant women at term, regardless of their parity[42]. In the 6 weeks following delivery, plasma and red cell folate return towards non-pregnant values, although lactation (which constitutes an added folate stress) may delay recovery[44].

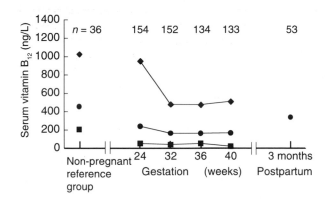

Figure 30. Serum vitamin B$_{12}$ levels (mean and range) measured longitudinally in pregnancy; only 53 of the original group had levels measured postpartum. Non-pregnant reference values were from 36 different women in their child-bearing years. *Data source*: ref. 45, with permission.

Comment: Serum vitamin B$_{12}$ levels fall in the first trimester[45]. They tend to be lower in smokers. Muscle and red cell vitamin B$_{12}$ concentrations also fall during pregnancy; however, vitamin B$_{12}$ absorption does not change[44].

Coagulation Factors

No. patients		41	48	47	66	62	48	61	61
Weeks		11–15	16–20	21–25	26–30	31–35	36–40	Post-delivery	Postnatal
Factor VII	Mean	111	129	150	158	162	171	134	94
	Range	60–206	68–244	80–280	75–332	84–312	87–336	70–255	52–171
Fibrinogen	Mean	3.63	3.65	3.65	3.78	4.17	4.23	4.61	2.65
(g/L)	Range	2.64–5.00	2.55–5.22	2.53–5.26	2.67–5.35	2.90–6.00	2.90–6.15	2.98–7.14	1.71–4.11
Factor X	Mean	103	111	115	126	123	127	117	90
	Range	62–169	74–166	74–177	78–203	78–194	72–208	72–191	54–149
Factor V	Mean	93	84	82	82	82	85	91	81
	Range	46–188	46–155	36–185	32–214	34–195	39–184	36–233	42–155
Factor II	Mean	125	128	125	124	115	115	112	106
	Range	70–224	75–218	73–214	79–193	74–179	68–194	74–170	68–165
Factor VIII:C	Mean	122	150	141	188	185	212	206	95
	Range	53–283	53–419	44–453	67–528	69–499	79–570	74–569	46–193
Factor VIII R: Ag	Mean	133	156	167	203	262	376	421	89
	Range	56–318	55–439	66–427	84–492	95–718	133–1064	169–1042	29–272
Factor VIIIR: Ag/VIII: C ratio	Mean	1.09	1.04	1.18	1.08	1.42	1.77	2.05	0.95
	Range	0.43–2.74	0.40–2.72	0.43–3.27	0.41–2.81	0.48–4.21	0.62–5.09	0.71–5.92	0.36–2.52

Figure 31. Coagulation factors (mean and 95% ranges) from a longitudinal study of 72 women (healthy primigravida, or multigravida whose previous pregnancies had been uncomplicated), aged 19–42 years. Post-delivery samples were taken between 6 hours and 4 days following delivery (mean 52 hours); postnatal samples were taken after 6 weeks. The postnatal samples yielded similar values to those from an age-matched non-pregnant group of women (*n*=66). *Data source*: ref. 46, with permission.

Comment: Normal pregnancy is a hypercoagulable state associated with increased levels of Factors VII, VIII and X, also a very marked increase in fibrinogen levels due to increased synthesis. Factor IX levels rise and Factor XI levels fall[44]. Not shown is the increase in fibrinopeptide A which occurs in the first trimester.

Naturally Occurring Anticoagulants and Fibrinolytic Factors

Naturally Occurring Anticoagulants and Fibrinolytic Factors

No. patients		41	48	47	66	62	48	61	61
Weeks		**11–15**	**16–20**	**21–25**	**26–30**	**31–35**	**36–40**	**Post-delivery**	**Postnatal**
FDPs (µg/mL)	Mean	1.07	1.06	1.09	1.13	1.28	1.32	1.66	1.04
		—	—	—	—	—	—	—	—
Fibrinolytic activity (Lysis time in hours)	Min	7.6	7.4	7.3	5.5	4.5	5.6	14.8	17.4
	Max	13.25	13.5	13.75	18.25	22.25	17.8	6.75	5.75
Antithrombin III: C	Mean	85	90	87	94	87	86	87	92
	Range	49–120	46–133	42–132	47–141	42–132	40–132	48–127	38–147
Antithrombin III: Ag	Mean	93	94	93	97	96	93	95	100
	Range	60–126	56–131	56–130	56–138	59–132	50–136	58–133	64–134
α_1– Antitrypsin	Mean	124	136	125	146	149	154	172	77
	Range	66–234	86–214	53–295	85–249	89–250	91–260	84–352	44–135
α_2– Macroglobulin	Mean	176	178	170	160	157	153	146	142
	Range	100–309	98–323	92–312	88–294	85–292	85–277	81–265	82–245

(Where no units are stated, values are expressed as percentage of standard.)

Figure 32. Naturally occurring anticoagulants and fibrinolytic factors (mean and 95% ranges), fibrinolytic activity (full range) and fibrin degradation products (mean values) from a longitudinal study. Patients were those described in Figure 31. *Data source*: ref. 46, with permission.

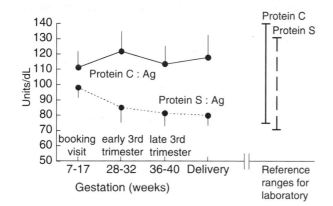

Figure 33. Protein S and C levels (mean and SD) from a longitudinal study in 14 healthy women aged 24–38 years. *Data source*: ref. 47, with permission.

Comment: Free protein S levels fall progressively during pregnancy but remain within the normal reference ranges; protein C levels change little. Antithrombin III levels are stable during pregnancy, fall in labor and then rise 1 week postpartum[44]. Fibrinolysis is depressed during pregnancy; both fibrinogen and plasminogen levels are elevated, but there are decreased levels of circulating plasminogen activator[48].

Complement System, Immune Complexes

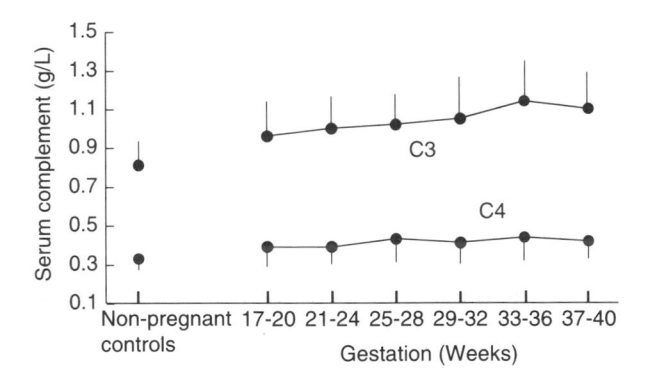

▲
Figure 34. Complement factors C3 and C4 (mean and SD) from a longitudinal study of 147 healthy women, who remained normotensive throughout pregnancy. The control population was 32 normal non-pregnant women, aged 15–41 years, 11 of whom were taking oral contraceptives. *Data source*: ref. 49, with permission.

Comment: Levels of C3 and C4 are significantly elevated during the second and third trimesters of pregnancy. Another cross-sectional study[50] showed elevated levels of C4, but not C3, during the first trimester. Circulating immune complexes are low during pregnancy[50]. There is some disagreement as to whether C3 degradation products are elevated[50] or normal[51]; no longitudinal studies have been done.

Markers of Inflammation

Erythrocyte sedimentation rate (ESR), C-reactive protein (CRP)

Comment: Values of ESR are high in pregnancy (typically > 30 mm in the first hour) due to elevated plasma globulins and fibrinogen[52]. Thus, ESR cannot be used as a marker for inflammation. Levels of C-reactive protein are undetectable in healthy pregnant women; elevations are due to intercurrent disease.

ENDOCRINOLOGY

Thyroid Function

Total thyroxine (T₄), tri-iodothyronine (T₃), T₃-uptake, thyroid binding globulin (TBG)

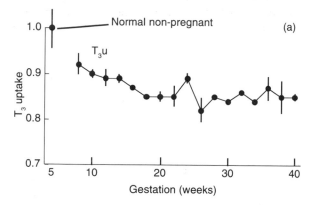

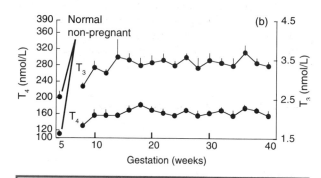

Figure 35. Total T₄, T₃ and T₃-uptake (mean ± SEM) from a mostly cross-sectional study of 339 women at various stages of pregnancy; 10–45 were sampled in each 2-week period from 6–40 weeks gestation. The controls were 40 non-pregnant women of similar age. *Data source*: ref. 53, with permission.

Comment: Serum total T_4 and T_3 concentrations are significantly elevated in pregnancy. The T_3 uptake test is low in pregnancy, indicating unsaturation of thyroid binding globulin (TBG). Thyroid binding globulin concentrations are doubled by the end of the first trimester, remain elevated throughout pregnancy, and fall slowly in the 6 weeks following delivery[54].

Thyroid Function

Free thyroxine (free T_4), free tri-iodothyronine (free T_3), thyroid stimulating hormone (TSH)

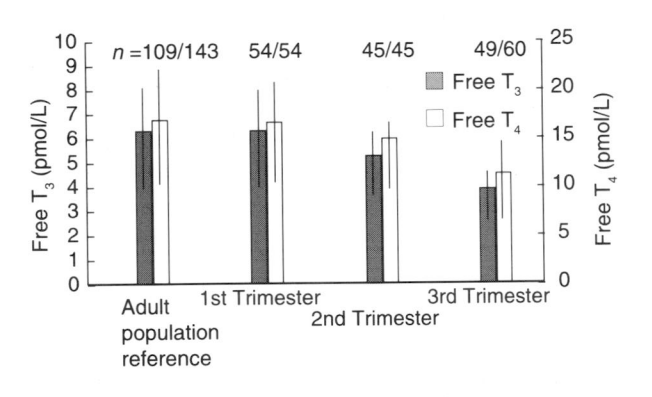

Figure 36. Free T_4 and T_3 concentrations (mean ± 2 SD) from a cross-sectional study of 159 women attending antenatal clinics; all were free from metabolic illness. The control samples were from 109 patients (male and female), taken from the routine workload of the laboratory (excluding those with thyroid disease, diabetes, cardiac disease, carcinoma, or patients in a postoperative state). *Data source*: ref. 55, with permission.

Comment: Free T_4 and T_3 concentrations in pregnancy, measured directly (rather than derived from resin uptake measurements) lie within normal non-pregnant ranges, generally[56]. However, a number of different assay methods are available; some yield lower values in late pregnancy[55]. TSH levels, measured by radioimmunoassay, are unchanged in normal pregnancy, although some studies have found low levels towards the end of the first trimester in association with the highest circulating concentrations of hCG[53].

Adrenal Function

Catecholamines

Figure 37. Adrenaline and noradrenaline concentrations (mean and SEM) from a longitudinal study of 52 women, mean age 28 years, who remained normotensive throughout pregnancy; 39 were primigravida. Samples were taken after 20 minutes rest in the left lateral position by venepuncture; a radioenzymic method was used for the assays. *Data source*: ref. 57, with permission.

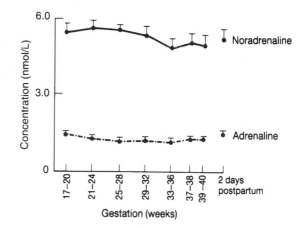

Comment: This study showed a decline in plasma levels of both adrenaline and noradrenaline as pregnancy progressed. Other studies (in which blood samples were taken from indwelling intravenous cannulae) have shown steady levels through pregnancy, with no difference between values during pregnancy and those in the early puerperium[58]. In healthy pregnant women, plasma noradrenaline and adrenaline show a diurnal pattern, with lowest levels during the night[59]. Urinary vanillomandelic acid (VMA) excretion has not been studied in healthy pregnancies, but is likely to be within the normal adult range.

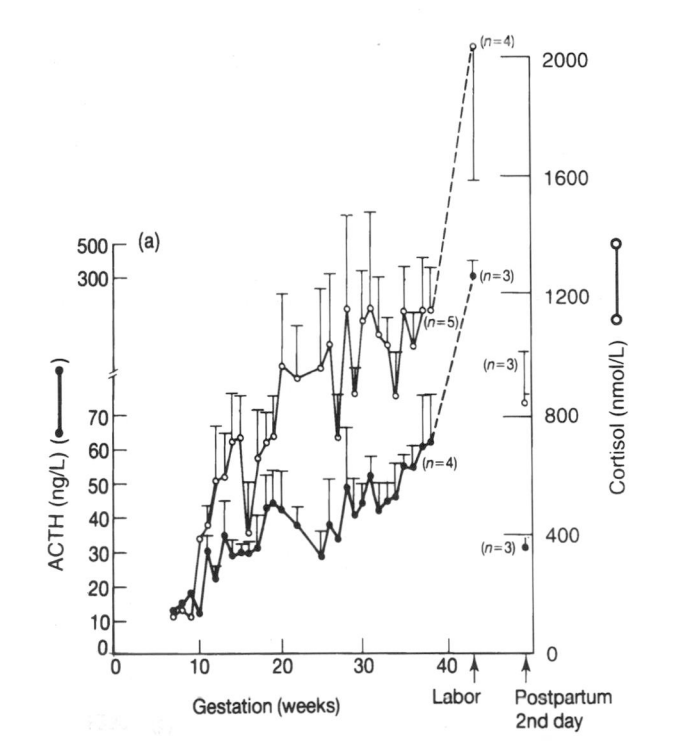

Glucocorticoids

Figure 38 (a) Adrenocorticotrophic hormone (ACTH) and cortisol concentrations (mean and SEM) from a longitudinal study of five healthy pregnant women, aged 17–28 years. Blood samples were taken weekly at 0800 to 0900 h after an overnight fast, from early pregnancy until delivery. Samples for ACTH measurement were collected improperly from one woman and had to be discarded. Samples were also taken from three of these subjects during labor and on the second postpartum day. *Data source*: ref. 60, with permission.

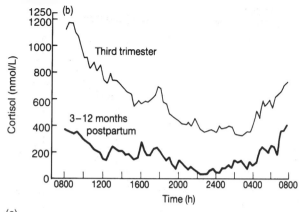

(b) Mean plasma cortisol throughout a 24-h study period from a study of seven primigravida in the third trimester and three non-pregnant women, two of whom had been studied during pregnancy. The non-pregnant women were at least 3 months after delivery and none was breast-feeding or using oral contraceptives. Samples were taken every 20 minutes. *Data source*: ref. 61, with permission.

(c)

	Plasma cortisol (nmol/L)			Free cortisol index	
	minimum	mean	maximum	minimum	maximum
	(in 24-h period)			(in 24-h period)	
Pregnant third trimester (*n*=7)	197 (25)	581 (28)	1206 (94)	2.2 (0.3)	15.7 (1.7)
Non-pregnant (*n*=3)	22 (6)	175 (25)	450 (3)	0.22 (0.05)	5.7 (0.9)

(c) Plasma cortisol and free cortisol index (mean and SD) from a study of seven primigravidae in the third trimester and three non-pregnant women, two of whom had been studied during pregnancy. Subjects were those described in Figure 38b. *Data source*: ref. 61, with permission.

Adrenal Function

Comment (Figure 38(a) – 38 (c)): Total plasma cortisol, free plasma cortisol and free cortisol index are increased in pregnancy as compared to the non-pregnant state. ACTH levels during pregnancy are variously reported as remaining within the normal range for non-pregnant subjects, increasing, or decreasing[60, 62], but there is agreement that levels rise with advancing gestation. The rise in ACTH during pregnancy is attributed to placental production of the peptide[62]. Normal diurnal patterns of cortisol (despite overall elevated levels) are found during pregnancy (i.e. lowest values at 2400 h, highest values at 0800 h[61]). The biological half-life of cortisol is increased in pregnancy[61]. Cortisol binding globulin (CBG) concentrations rise steadily during pregnancy, reaching twice normal values by mid-gestation[63]. Cortisol production rate during pregnancy has been described as being depressed[64] or elevated[61]. Urinary free cortisol more than doubles during pregnancy[65]. Plasma cortisol levels measured at 0800 h following 1 mg of dexamethasone given orally at 2300 h the previous evening suppress to < 5 μg/dL (a normal response)[66]; however, urinary cortisol levels do not suppress as much in pregnant as in non-pregnant subjects[62]. The cortisol response to an ACTH challenge (Synacthen test) is unchanged in pregnancy[67].

Prolactin

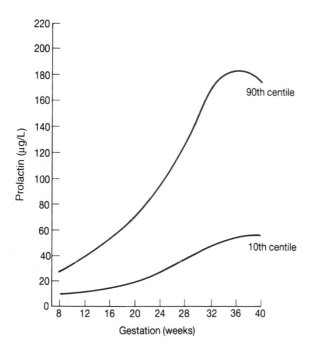

Figure 39. Serum prolactin (10th and 90th centiles) from a mostly cross-sectional study of 839 women with uncomplicated singleton pregnancies between 8 and 40 weeks gestation; a total of 980 blood samples were taken. All samples were collected between 0900 and 1100 h. Any woman who developed a pregnancy complication was rejected from the normal series. *Data source*: ref. 68, with permission.

Comment: Prolactin concentrations increase 10–20-fold during the course of pregnancy. There is a normal circadian rhythm, with a nocturnal rise[69]. In labor, there is an acute fall in levels, then a postpartum surge during the first 2 hours following delivery[70]; these changes are not seen in women undergoing elective cesarean deliveries. Prolactin levels approach the normal range 2–3 weeks after delivery in non-lactating women, but remain elevated in those who breast-feed their infants[71].

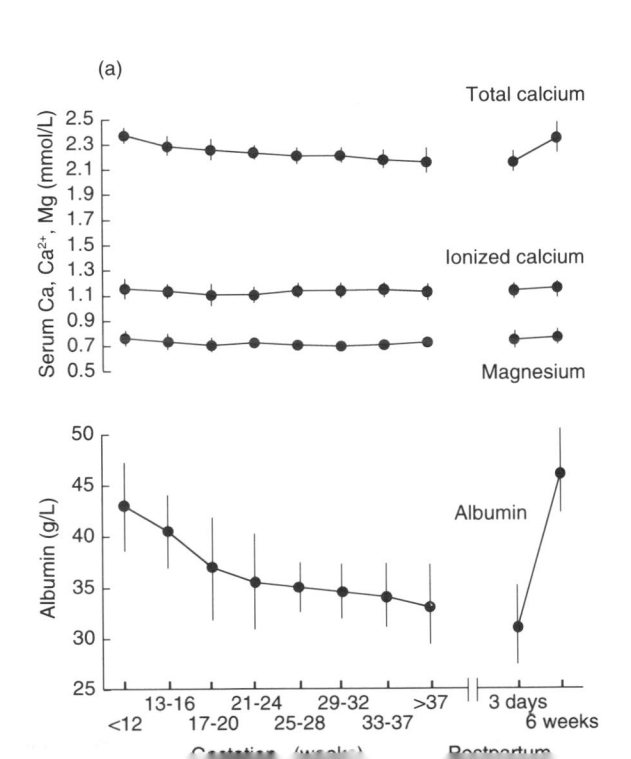

Calcium Metabolism

Total and ionized calcium, magnesium, albumin, parathyroid hormone (PTH), calcitonin, vitamin D

Figure 40. (a) Total and ionized calcium, magnesium and albumin (mean ± SD) from a longitudinal study of 30 women, recruited in the first trimester and studied at 4-week intervals. Samples were also taken on the third postpartum day and during the sixth postpartum week. The subjects ranged in age from 19–33 years; 20 were primigravidae. Samples were collected by venepuncture after an overnight fast. (Calcium, mmol/L × 4 = mg/dL; magnesium, mmol/L × 2.4 = mg/dL.) *Data source*: ref. 72, with permission.

(b)

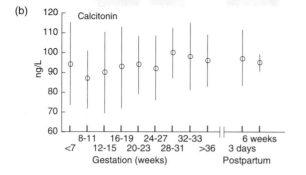

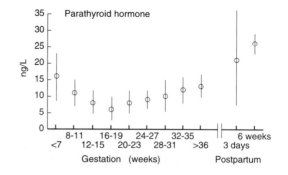

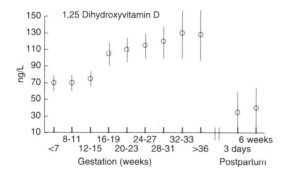

(b) Calcitonin, parathyroid hormone and 1,25 dihydroxy-vitamin D (mean ± SD) from a longitudinal study of 20 women, aged 22–34 years, 12 of whom were nulli-parous. All had uncomplicated pregnancies of more than 38 weeks gestation. The only medication they received was ferrous sulfate. Blood samples were taken in the morning after an overnight fast. Samples were collected at 4-week intervals, the first being taken before 7 weeks gestation; also on the third postpartum day and during the sixth postpartum week. *Data source*: ref. 73, with permission.

Comment (Figure 40 (a) and (b)): Total serum calcium declines during pregnancy, in association with the fall in serum albumin; however, ionized calcium levels remain constant. Serum intact PTH levels are lower in pregnancy than at 6 weeks postpartum; they reach their nadir in mid-pregnancy. A menstrual cyclicity in PTH has also been noted, with higher values corresponding to times of increased estrogen secretion[72]. Calcitonin levels are not significantly altered in pregnancy. 1,25 Dihydroxyvitamin D levels rise with advancing gestation and are significantly higher than during the puerperium. Some 1α-hydroxylation of 25 hydroxyvitamin D has been demonstrated in the placenta to account for this rise and the consequent suppression of PTH[73].

Placental Biochemistry

Serum alpha fetoprotein (SAFP)

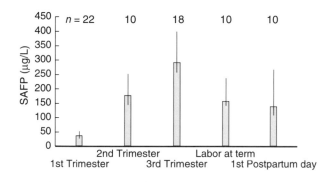

Figure 41. Serum alpha fetoprotein (median and IQ range) from a cross-sectional study, although samples from women in labor and on the first postpartum day were paired. SAFP was measured by radioimmunoassay. *Data source*: ref. 74, with permission.

Comment: In the second trimester, SAFP rises by approximately 15% per week[75]. Reference ranges for SAFP in the second trimester are established by individual screening laboratories for their own population and are usually expressed as multiples of the median (MoM) for gestation. Twin pregnancies are associated with SAFP levels approximately twice as high as those of singleton pregnancies[75]. Maternal weight is inversely related to SAFP levels, probably due to the dilutional effect of a larger vascular compartment[75].

Placental Biochemistry

Human chorionic gonadotrophin (hCG)

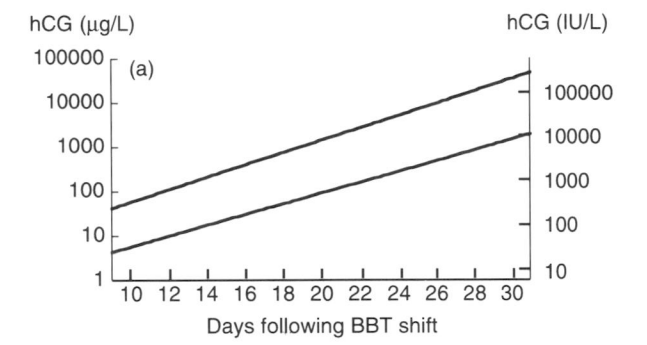

Figure 42. (a) Serum values of the ß-subunit of hCG (95% CI) measured in 189 women who subsequently had successful pregnancies (total of 280 samples analyzed). They were patients in an infertility clinic and were keeping basal body temperature (BBT) charts to indicate the timing of ovulation. Some conceptions were spontaneous; other patients were treated with clomiphene citrate, human menopausal gonadotrophin and/or hCG (a single injection of 5000 IU to induce ovulation). A radioimmunoassay was used for ß-hCG. *Data source*: ref. 76, with permission. (b) Total serum hCG (mean ± SD) from a longitudinal study of 20 healthy women. The first samples were drawn as early in pregnancy as possible, with subsequent samples every 3–4 weeks; the last sample was taken during labor. Samples were classified into groups with a class interval of 30 days. hCG was determined by radioimmunoassay; the international hCG standard was used as a reference. *Data source*: ref. 77, with permission.

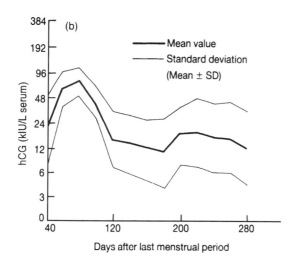

(b)

Comment: The mean doubling time of ß-hCG is 2.2 days ± 1.0 (2 SD)[76]. Low hCG values which do not double within this range are associated with ectopic pregnancies or spontaneous abortions[76]. Women with male fetuses have significantly lower hCG levels than do those with female fetuses[77].

Human placental lactogen (hPL)

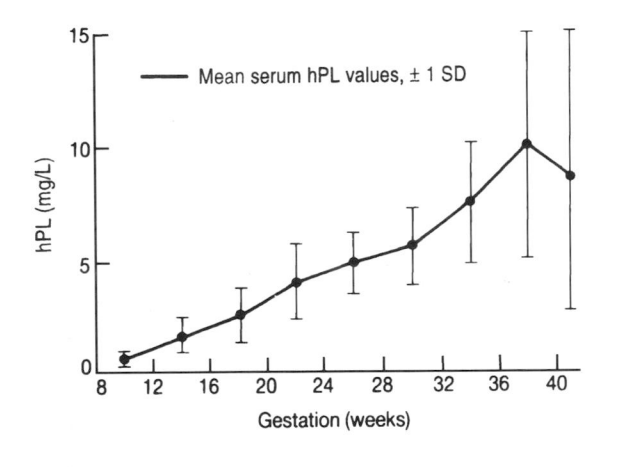

Figure 43. Serum hPL values (mean ± SD) from a cross-sectional study of 151 normal women with singleton pregnancies attending the antenatal clinic. hPL was measured by radioimmunoassay. *Data source*: ref. 78, with permission.

Comment: hPL levels in women with multiple pregnancies are outside these ranges; however, if values are corrected for predicted placental weight then they are appropriate for gestational age[78]. Four hours after delivery of the placenta, plasma hPL is virtually undetectable; the half-life of hPL in the plasma is 21–23 minutes[79].

Estriol (E₃)

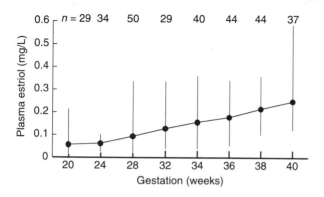

Figure 44. Plasma estriol (mean and range) from a cross-sectional study in women with uncomplicated pregnancies. Plasma estriol was measured by a fluorometric method. *Data source*: ref. 80, with permission.

Comment: The normal range of plasma estriol in pregnancy is wide. In order to assess the significance of values outside this range, trends should be studied over several days.

FETAL VALUES

PHYSIOLOGY

Early Embryonic Structures

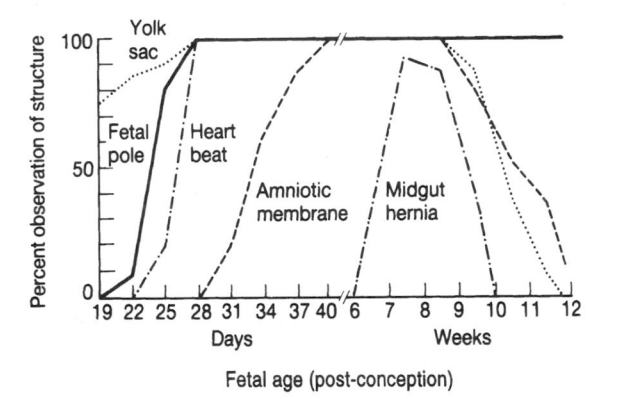

Figure 45. Visualization by ultrasound of yolk sac, fetal pole, heart beat, amniotic membrane, midgut hernia from a longitudinal study of 39 women with known dates of ovulation; most were patients from an assisted conception unit. They were scanned using a vaginal probe weekly, once pregnancy had been confirmed, starting as early as 18 days post-conception. Five subjects had twin pregnancies. *Data source*: ref. 81, with permission.

Comment: Transvaginal ultrasound scanning yields better images in the first trimester than does transabdominal scanning. By 28 days post-conception, fetal viability may be confirmed by visualization of a heart beat. The fetal heart rate increases from 90 bpm to 145 bpm by 7 weeks post-conception[81].

Biometry

Crown–rump length (CRL)

Figure 46. Crown–rump length (mean ± 2 SD) from a cross-sectional study of 334 women who were certain of the date of their last menstrual periods (LMP) and had normal regular menstrual cycles. The study covered the time period from 6 to 14 weeks post-LMP. A trans-abdominal ultrasound technique was used and the longest length of fetal echoes was found and measured. *Data source*: ref. 82, with permission.

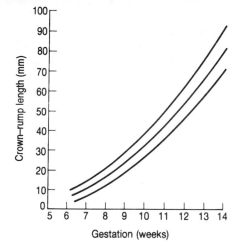

Comment: CRL measurements can only be used effectively in the first trimester. Other studies have found very similar values for CRL; measurements are not influenced by maternal age, height or parity[83]. In a smaller, longitudinal study CRL was found to be significantly smaller in female than male fetuses[83]. No differences have been found in CRL measurements between Asian and European patients[84].

Biparietal diameter (BPD)

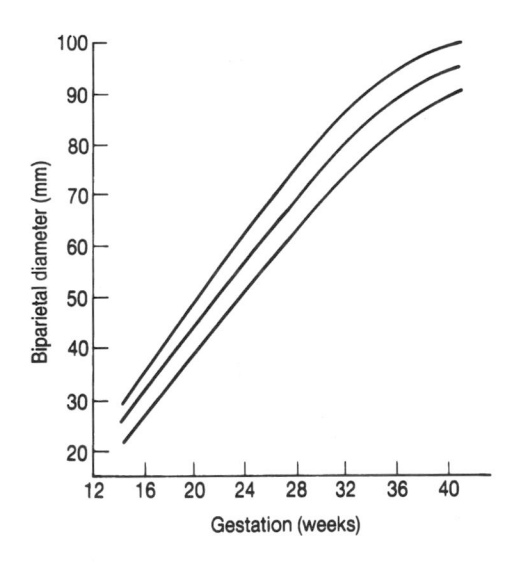

Figure 47. Biparietal diameter (mean ± 2 SD) from a longitudinal study of 41 women with regular menstruation and a known last menstrual period (LMP). They were scanned every 2–4 weeks, beginning 13–14 weeks post-LMP; in total 493 scans were performed. *Data source*: ref. 85, with permission.

Comment: Other studies have found similar values for BPD[84,86]. No differences in BPD measurements have been found between Asian and European patients living in the same city[84].

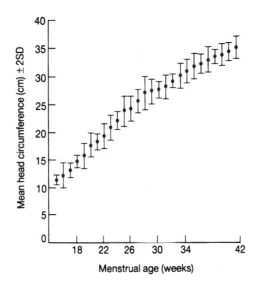

Figure 48. Head circumference (mean ± 2 SD) from a cross-sectional study of 400 consecutive healthy patients who had certain menstrual dates and singleton pregnancies: most were middle-class Caucasians. *Data source*: ref. 87, with permission.

Comment: HC measurements are particularly useful in the assessment of gestational age when there is an abnormality of fetal head shape, e.g. dolicocephaly.

Abdominal circumference (AC)

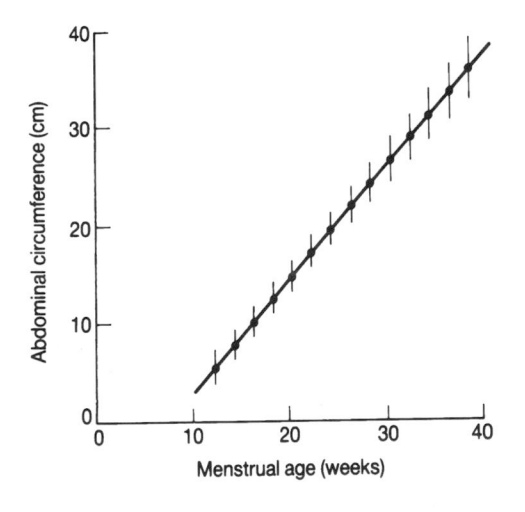

Figure 49. Abdominal circumference (mean ± SD) from a longitudinal study of 20 women with certain last menstrual periods (LMP); most were patients in an infertility programme. They were scanned every 3 weeks, beginning 14–16 weeks post-LMP. *Data source*: ref. 88, with permission.

Comment: Another study of fetal AC measurements suggests that there is a flattening off of growth towards term[89]. Some of the discrepancies between studies are due to different mathematical curve-fitting techniques applied to the experimental data, as well as to differences in the design of studies and numbers of subjects involved[88,90].

Femur length (FL)

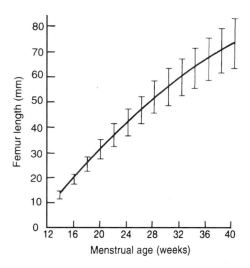

Figure 50. Femur length (regression line and 95% CI) from a cross-sectional study of 254 women between 13 and 39 weeks gestation; all were certain of the dates of their last menstrual periods and had regular cycles. Ultrasound scans were performed transabdominally using a 2.4 or 3.5 MHz transducer. The longest image of the femur was measured in a straight line with the transducer along the long axis of the femur (to avoid foreshortening). *Data source*: ref. 91, with permission.

Comment: The rate of growth of the femur decreases with advancing gestational age, but the variability increases[91]. Another study from a different geographical location found very similar values for FL in pregnancy[92].

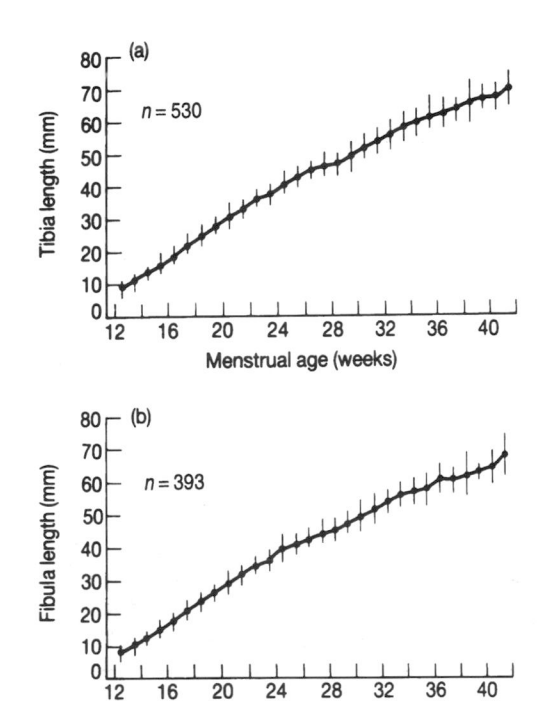

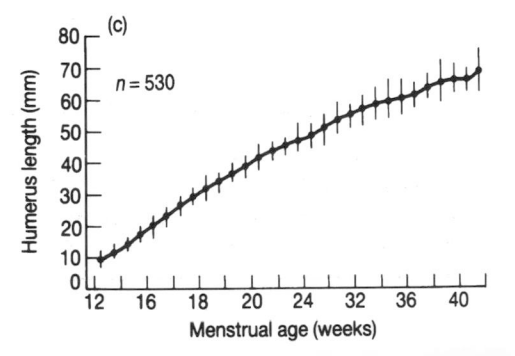

Limb bone lengths

◀ **Figure 51**. Lengths of (a) tibia, (b) fibula, (c) humerus, (d) radius, and (e) ulna (mean ± 2SD) from a cross-sectional study of 530 healthy women between 13 and 42 weeks gestation. Menstrual age was confirmed in each case by an early ultrasound scan to measure CRL. Lengths of the tibia, humerus and radius were measured in every case, but those of the fibula and ulna in 339 cases. *Data source*: ref. 93, with permission. ▼

Comment: All limb bones show linear growth from 13–25 weeks; thereafter the growth is non-linear. Good agreement has been found between ultrasound and X-ray measurements of limb bones. Tables are available to allow assessment of gestational age from measurement of limb bone lengths[94]. This use of limb bone measurements should be distinguished from tables or graphs of normal measurements at known gestational age which allow assessment of possible skeletal dysplasias[93,95].

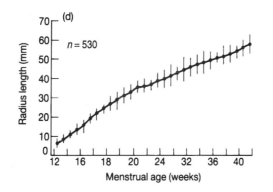

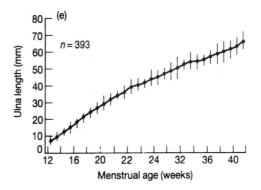

Foot

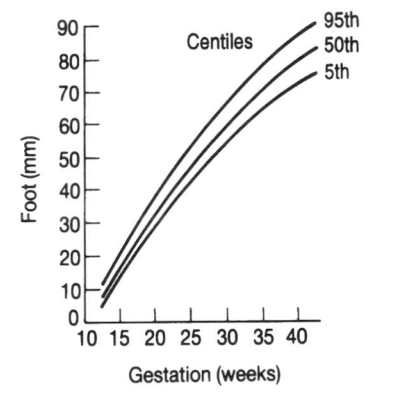

Figure 52. Length of foot (5th, 50th and 95th centiles) from a cross-sectional study of 669 healthy women with singleton pregnancies; any who subsequently delivered an infant with a significant malformation, abnormal karyotype, or other disease was excluded from the analysis. All women had a known last menstrual period and there was agreement between menstrual age and ultrasound dating (at the time of the initial scan). Approximately 20 measurements were obtained for each variable for each week of pregnancy from 12 until 42 weeks gestation. *Data source*: ref. 86, with permission.

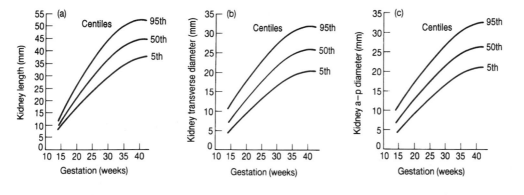

Comment: The ratio of the transverse renal circumference to the abdominal circumference (in a section at the level of the umbilical vein) is a simple way of assessing normal kidney size; values are 0.27–0.30 from 17 weeks until term[96].

Figure 53. Kidney measurements (5th, 50th and 95th centiles) from a cross-sectional study of 669 healthy women with singleton pregnancies; all had a known last menstrual period and there was agreement between menstrual age and ultrasound dating (at the time of the initial scan). Approximately 20 measurements were obtained for each variable for each week of pregnancy from 12 until 42 weeks gestation. *Data source*: ref. 86, with permission.

Orbital diameters

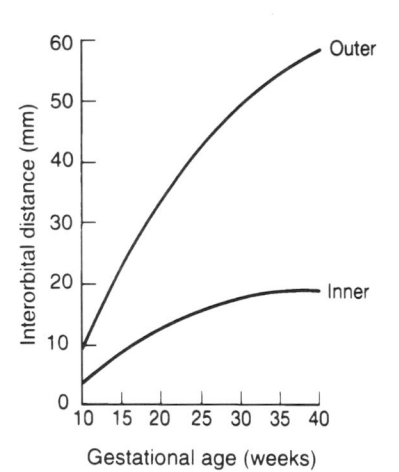

Figure 54. Interorbital distance (mean) from a cross-sectional study of 180 healthy women from 22–40 weeks gestation. A scan plane was obtained which transected the occiput, orbits and nasal processes. *Data source*: ref. 97, with permission.

Comment: Outer-orbital diameter (IOD) is closely related to biparietal diameter (BPD). It is a useful measurement when the fetal position precludes accurate measurement of BPD.

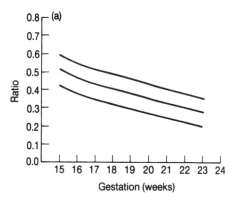

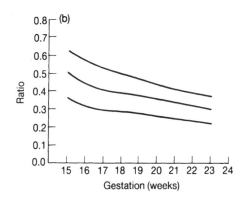

Figure 55. Ventricular ratios (mean ± 2 SD) from a cross-sectional study of 101 women in the second trimester. The ratio of the distance from the lateral border of the frontal horn of the lateral cerebral ventricle to the midline echo compared to the hemispheric width at the same axial scan plane was computed as the anterior VH ratio (a). Similarly, the posterior VH ratio (b) was calculated from measurements of the temporal horn of the lateral ventricle. *Data source*: ref. 98, with permission.

Comment: The most reliable measurements of the ventricular system are made using the frontal horns of the lateral cerebral ventricles as they are the easiest to identify. As a general rule, ventricular diameter should be less than 10 mm.

Biometry

PHYSIOLOGY

Cerebellum

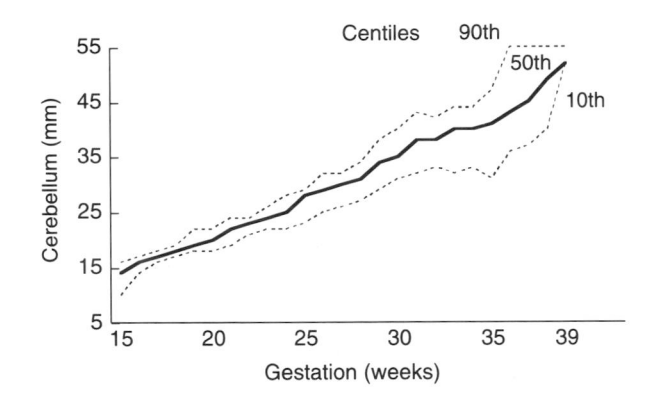

Figure 56. Cerebellar diameter (10th, 50th and 90th centiles) from a cross-sectional study of 371 normal pregnant women of gestational age 13–40 weeks. In all women, gestational age was confirmed by ultrasonography before 14 weeks. The transverse cerebellar diameter was measured in an axial scan plane through the posterior fossa. *Data source*: ref. 99, with permission.

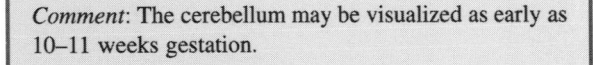

Comment: The cerebellum may be visualized as early as 10–11 weeks gestation.

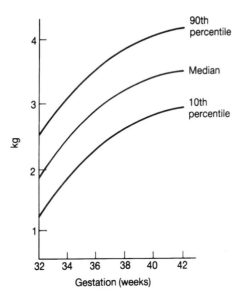

Figure 57. Birth weight (10th, 50th and 90th centiles) from analysis of 46,703 singleton births in Aberdeen, Scotland, between 1948 and 1964. Most of the mothers were of Caucasian origin and were themselves born in Scotland. *Data source*: ref. 100, with permission.

Comment: Birth weight ranges by gestational age need to be established for different populations, as they are influenced by ethnic, socio-economic and geographic factors, etc.[101] Different ranges apply to infants from multiple pregnancies.

Biometry

Weight estimated from ultrasound measurements

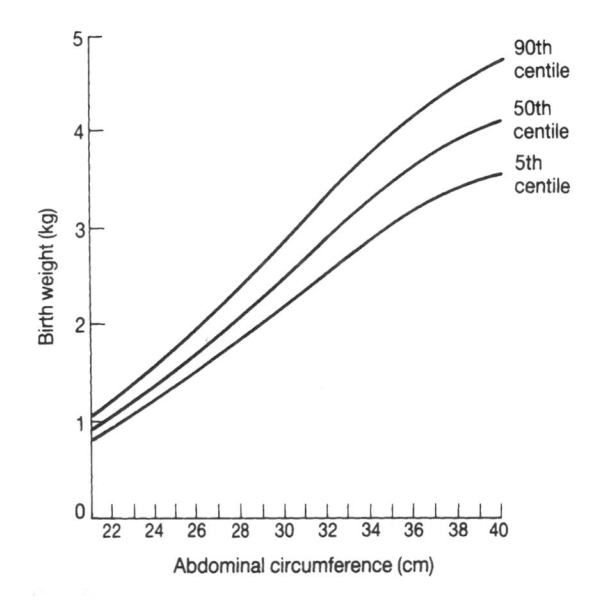

Figure 58. Weight estimated from ultrasound measurements (5th, 50th and 90th centiles) from a study of 138 women, who had an ultrasound examination within 48 hours of delivery for the measurement of fetal abdominal circumference (AC). The actual birth weights were compared with the AC measurements and a polynomial equation derived to describe the relationship. *Data source*: ref. 102, with permission.

Comment: Equations have also been derived for estimating fetal weight from various combinations of ultrasonic measurements (AC, BPD, HC, FL)[103,104] which are claimed to be more accurate than those based on AC measurements alone.

Amniotic Fluid

Total volume

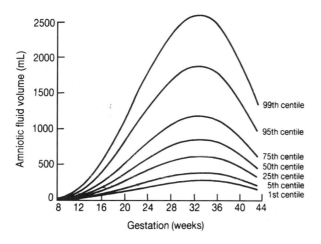

Figure 59. Total amniotic fluid volume (1st, 5th, 25th, 50th, 75th, 95th and 99th centiles). Composite analysis of 12 published reports of amniotic fluid volume in human pregnancy, totaling 705 measurements. Amniotic fluid volumes were either measured directly at the time of hysterotomy or indirectly using an indicator dilution technique. Only healthy pregnancies were included; any complicated by fetal death or anomaly, or by maternal disease were excluded. *Data source*: ref. 105, with permission.

Amniotic fluid index (AFI)

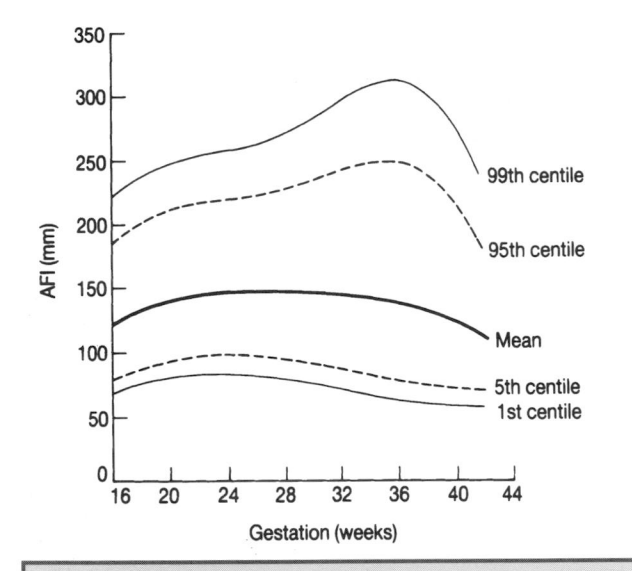

Figure 60. Amniotic fluid index (1st, 5th, 50th, 95th and 99th centiles) from a prospective study of 791 patients. Any who did not have a normal pregnancy outcome (i.e. infant born at term, between 10th and 90th centile for birth weight, with 5-minute Apgar score above 6, and without congenital anomaly) were subsequently excluded. Ultrasound imaging was performed and the uterus divided into four quadrants along the sagittal midline and midway up the fundus. Amniotic fluid index was calculated as the sum of the deepest vertical dimension (in millimeters) of the amniotic fluid pocket in each quadrant of the uterus. *Data source*: ref. 106, with permission.

Comment: Amniotic fluid volume rises to a plateau between 22 and 39 weeks gestation of 700–850 mL. This corresponds to an AFI of 140–150 mm. After term, there is a significant decline in amniotic fluid volume.

Pressure

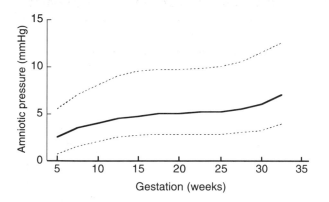

Figure 61. Amniotic fluid pressure (mean and 95% CI) from a cross-sectional study of 171 singleton pregnancies, subsequently shown to have normal karyotype, in whom amniotic fluid volume was subjectively assessed as normal on ultrasonic appearances. All patients were scheduled to undergo a transamniotic invasive procedure for diagnostic reasons or else were to undergo therapeutic termination of pregnancy. Amniotic fluid pressure was measured using a manometry technique referenced to the top of the maternal abdomen. *Data source*: ref. 107, with permission.

Comment: Amniotic fluid pressure rises with gestation, although there is a mid-trimester plateau of 4–5 mmHg. Pressure was not influenced by parity or maternal age and was similar in twin and singleton pregnancies[107].

Amniotic Fluid

Osmolality

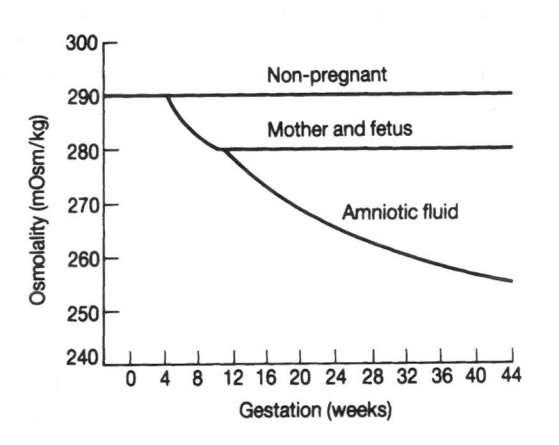

Figure 62. Amniotic fluid osmolality (mean) from a composite analysis of six published reports of amniotic fluid osmolality. *Data source*: ref. 108, with permission.

Comment: In early pregnancy the composition of amniotic fluid is consistent with a transudate of maternal or fetal plasma[109]. The fetal skin becomes keratinized by mid-pregnancy and the amniotic fluid solute concentrations decrease as fetal urine becomes more dilute[109]. Thus there is an osmotic gradient between amniotic fluid and both maternal and fetal plasma.

Cardiovascular Indices

Ductus venosus Doppler indices

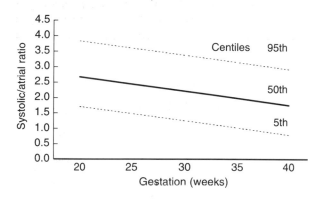

Figure 63. Systolic:atrial ratio from ductus venosus Doppler flow-velocity waveforms. These were recorded in a cross-sectional study of 164 appropriate-for-gestational age fetuses at 16–42 weeks of gestation, who did not have structural or chromosomal abnormalities. Velocity waveforms were recorded from the ductus venosus at its origin from the umbilical vein as visualized in a transverse section of the fetal abdomen with a color and pulsed Doppler machine. The angle of insonation of the vessel was kept low; any recordings where this angle exceeded 20° were rejected. The ductus venosus waveforms were recognized by their characteristic biphasic pattern. The ratio between peak systolic velocity and that occurring during atrial contraction (the nadir of the waveform) was calculated. *Data source*: ref. 110, with permission.

Comment: Color-flow mapping Doppler equipment is necessary for the correct identification of the ductus venosus; waveforms from the intrahepatic portion of the umbilical vein and the inferior vena cava are different. The declining systolic:atrial ratio is interpreted as indicating a relative increase in blood flow during end diastole, i.e. improved cardiac filling.

Cardiovascular Indices

Umbilical artery Doppler indices

◀ **Figure 64**. Doppler indices from umbilical artery flow-velocity waveforms (mean ± 2 SD). They were obtained in a longitudinal study of 15 normal pregnancies scanned every 2 weeks from 24–28 weeks gestation until delivery, eight of whom had been recruited at 16 weeks and also scanned every 4 weeks through the second trimester. In all subjects gestational age had been confirmed by ultrasound scanning at 16 weeks gestation. A range-gated pulsed Doppler beam was guided from the ultrasound image to insonate the umbilical artery. (a) Resistance (Pourcelot) Index ($[A-B] \div A$), (b) Pulsatility Index ($[A-B] \div M$) and (c) A/B Ratio ($A \div B$) were calculated (where A=maximum systolic frequency, B=maximum diastolic frequency, M=mean frequency as measured from the Doppler-shift waveforms). *Data source*: ref. 111, with kind permission from Elsevier Science Ireland Ltd, Co. Clare, Ireland.

▼

Comment: After 16 weeks gestation there is forward flow in umbilical arteries throughout the cardiac cycle, as evidenced by positive Doppler-shift frequencies even at the end of diastole. Declining values of Resistance Index, Pulsatility Index and A/B Ratio with gestation are interpreted as indicating decreasing resistance in the placental circulation.

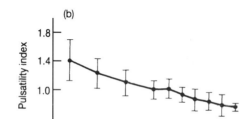

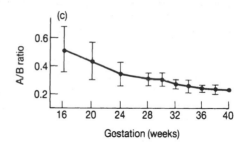

Cardiovascular Indices

Cardiac output

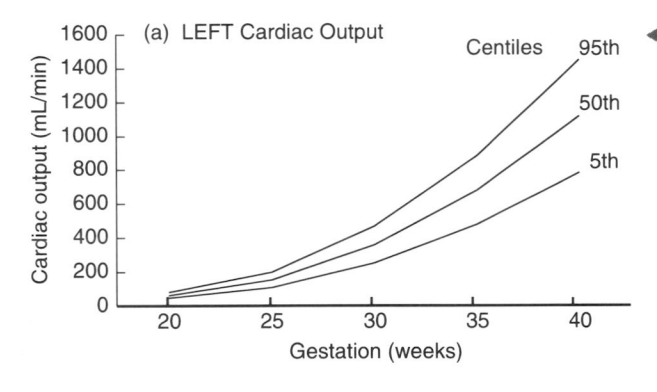

◀ **Figure 65**. (a) Left cardiac output (LCO) and (b) right cardiac output (RCO) calculated at the level of the outflow tracts (5th, 50th, 95th centiles) from a longitudinal study of 26 healthy, singleton fetuses studied at weekly intervals. Velocity waveforms were recorded from the ascending aorta and pulmonary artery with the flow parallel to the Doppler beam; any recordings obtained with the beam angle > 20° were rejected. Valve diameter measurements were made from video tape images; valve areas were calculated by assuming a circular cross-section. *Data source*: ref. 112, with permission.

▼

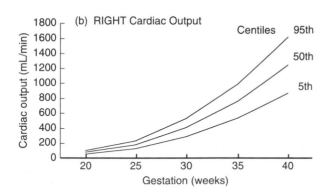

(b) RIGHT Cardiac Output

Centiles

95th

50th

5th

Cardiac output (mL/min) — Gestation (weeks)

Comment: Cardiac output rises progressively with gestation, RCO being slightly higher than LCO (RCO/LCO ratio approximately 1.3). Peak flow velocity at both aortic and pulmonary valves rises with gestation. This is attributed to progressive improvement in cardiac contractility, reduction in afterload and increase in preload[112]. Calculations of volume flow like these in fetal vessels are prone to high coefficients of variation as any error in the measurement of diameter (e.g. valve ring diameter) is further magnified as cross-sectional area is computed.

Cardiovascular Indices

Umbilical venous pressure (UVP)

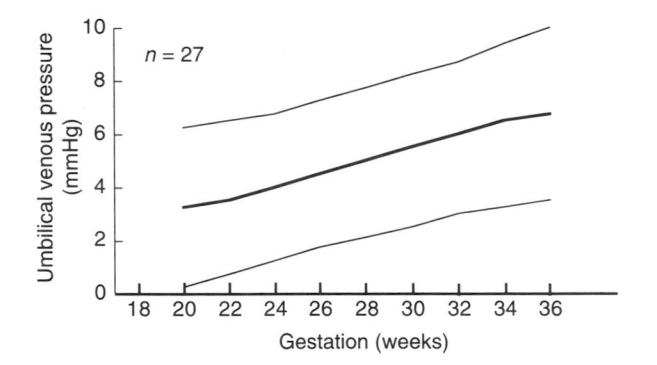

Figure 66. Umbilical venous pressure (mean and 95% CI) from 27 fetuses referred for assessment of possible intrauterine infection or hemolysis, but subsequently shown to be unaffected. They all underwent cordocentesis and after the necessary blood samples had been obtained the needle was connected to a pressure transducer. The transducer was placed at the level of the fetal heart and the pressure read at its nadir. The needle was confirmed to be in the umbilical vein by the non-pulsatile pressure tracing obtained and by observing the direction of flow of injected saline. As the needle was withdrawn, the amniotic cavity pressure was recorded. Umbilical venous pressure was calculated by subtracting amniotic pressure from the measured umbilical venous pressure. *Data source*: ref. 113, with permission.

Comment: Umbilical venous pressure rises with advancing gestation, but remains within a narrow range. Values above the CI are associated with cardiac failure[114].

Mean umbilical arterial pressure (MAP)

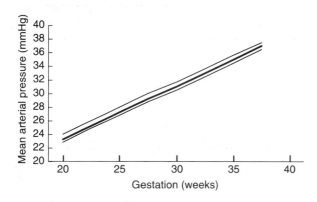

Figure 67. Mean umbilical arterial pressure (mean and 95% CI) from 30 normal fetuses. These had been referred for assessment of possible infection or hemolysis but were found to be unaffected. The methodology was identical to that outlined in Figure 66. It was apparent that the needle tip was in an umbilical artery rather than vein (due to a pulsatile pressure signal). *Data source*: ref. 115, with permission.

Comment: The normal range of arterial pressure in the fetus is very narrow (much more so than for umbilical venous pressure). Arterial pressure rises as gestational age increases.

Cardiovascular Indices

Fetal heart rate (FHR)

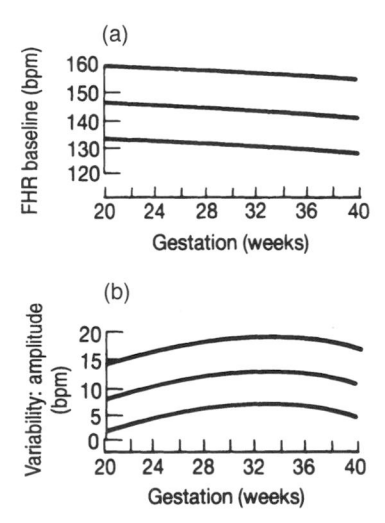

(a)

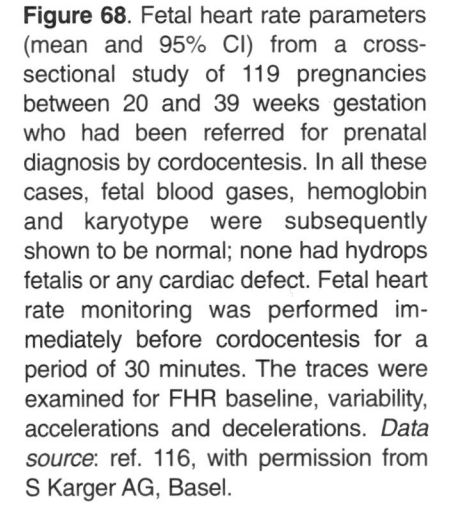

(b)

Figure 68. Fetal heart rate parameters (mean and 95% CI) from a cross-sectional study of 119 pregnancies between 20 and 39 weeks gestation who had been referred for prenatal diagnosis by cordocentesis. In all these cases, fetal blood gases, hemoglobin and karyotype were subsequently shown to be normal; none had hydrops fetalis or any cardiac defect. Fetal heart rate monitoring was performed immediately before cordocentesis for a period of 30 minutes. The traces were examined for FHR baseline, variability, accelerations and decelerations. *Data source*: ref. 116, with permission from S Karger AG, Basel.

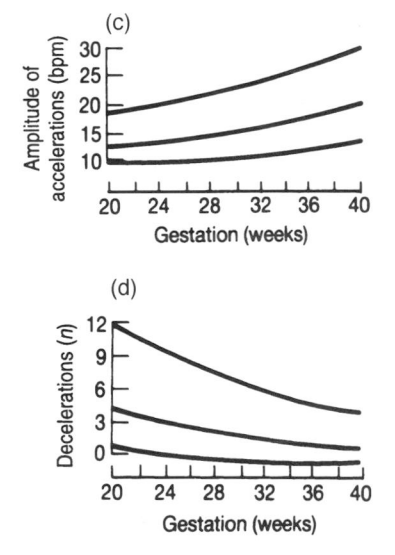

(c)

(d)

- At least two accelerations (>15 beats for >15 s) in 20 min, baseline heart rate 110–150 bpm, baseline variability 5–25 bpm, absence of decelerations.

- Sporadic decelerations amplitude <40 bpm are acceptable if duration <15 s, or <30 s following an acceleration.

- When there is moderate tachycardia (150–170 bpm) or bradycardia (100–110 bpm) a reactive trace is reassuring of good health.

Figure 69. Features of a normal antepartum cardiotocogram (non-stress test). *Data source*: ref. 117, with permission.

Comment: Baseline FHR decreases with gestation, but the variability of the baseline increases. The number and amplitude of accelerations increase with gestation. Spontaneous decelerations are commonly found in the second trimester and early third trimester, but rarely in healthy fetuses approaching term. During labor, criteria for the interpretation of FHR traces alter (see Figure 83).

Cardiovascular Indices

Biophysical profile score (BPS)

Fetal variable	Normal behavior (score = 2)	Abnormal behavior (score = 0)
Fetal breathing movements	More than 1 episode of 30 s duration, intermittent within a 30 min overall period. Hiccups count. (Not continuous throughout the observation time)	Repetitive or continuous breathing without cessation. Completely absent breathing or no sustained episodes
Gross body/limb movements	Three or more discrete body/limb movements in a 30 min period. Continuous active movement episodes are considered as a single movement. Also included are fine motor movements, positional adjustments and so on	Two or fewer body/limb movements in a 30 min observation period
Fetal tone and posture	Demonstration of active extension with rapid return of flexion of fetal limbs, brisk repositioning/trunk rotation. Opening and closing of hand, mouth, kicking, etc.	Only low-velocity movements, incomplete return to flexion, flaccid extremity positions; abnormal fetal posture. Includes score = 0 when FM absent
Fetal heart rate reactivity	Greater than 2 significant accelerations associated with maternally palpated fetal movement during a 20 min cardiotocogram. (Accelerations graded for gestation: 10 beats/min for 10 s before 26 weeks; 15 beats/min for 15 s after 26 weeks; 20 beats/min for 20 s at term)	Fetal movement and accelerations not coupled. Insufficient accelerations, absent accelerations, or decelerative trace. Mean variation <20 on numerical analysis of CTG
Amniotic fluid volume evaluation	One pocket of >3 cm without umbilical cord loops. More than 1 pocket of >2cm without cord loops. No elements of subjectively reduced amniotic volume	No cord-free pocket >2 cm, or elements of subjectively reduced amniotic fluid volume definite

Figure 70. Scoring system for five fetal biophysical variables (breathing movements, gross body/limb movements, tone/posture, heart rate reactivity and amniotic fluid volume) developed for the assessment of patients with high-risk pregnancies. This scoring system was evaluated in 216 patients who were studied in the week prior to delivery and whose eventual pregnancy outcome was documented. No perinatal deaths occurred in this study when all five variables were present at the time of examination with ultrasound and cardiotocography. Low scores (≤6 out of 10) were associated with increased incidence of adverse outcomes (fetal distress in labor, Apgar scores ≤ 7 at 5 minutes of age, perinatal death). *Data source*: ref. 118, with permission.

Comment: Various means of monitoring fetal well-being antenataly have been proposed (cardiotocography, observation of fetal breathing patterns, measurement of amniotic fluid volume); however, scoring systems which take into consideration a combination of behavioral parameters are superior in their ability to detect a compromised fetus and hence to allow its early delivery[119]. This has led to improvement in perinatal mortality rates, even in a high-risk group of pregnant women[119]. It must be borne in mind that fetal behavior is periodic and affected by external factors (e.g. maternal ingestion of stimulant or depressant drugs, maternal hypo- or hyperglycemia) and by structural or genetic abnormalities of the fetus. Fetal behavior abruptly changes from a quiescent to an active pattern and *vice versa*, thus ultrasound observation may need to be extended for 30 or 40 minutes to confirm absence of fetal movements or breathing; most BPS studies are completed in less than 10 minutes[118]. Acute disasters may occur which invalidate the predictive accuracy of the BPS, (e.g. abruptio placentae, diabetic ketoacidosis, eclampsia).

BIOCHEMISTRY

Proteins

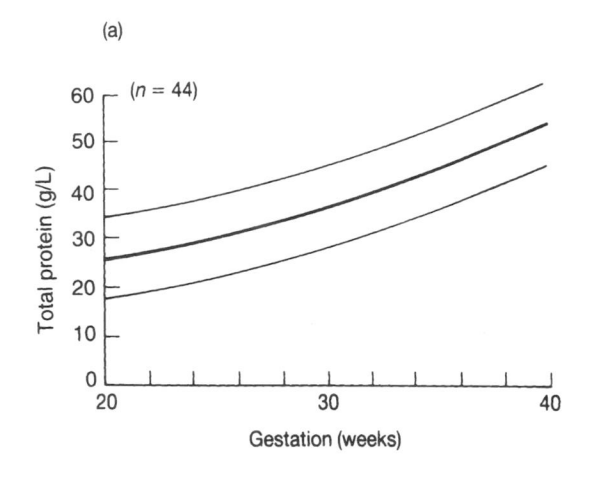

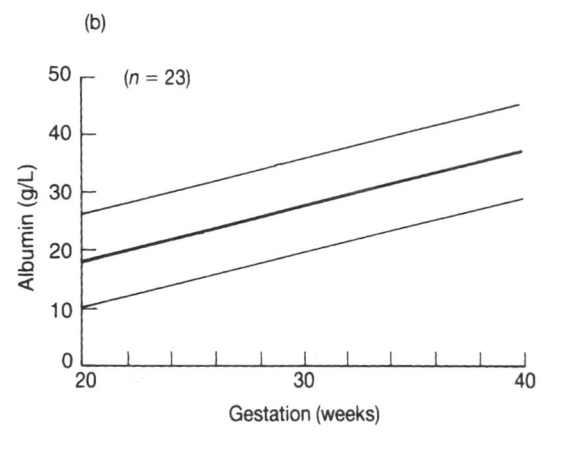

Figure 71. Total protein and albumin concentrations (regression curve and 95% CI) from a cross-sectional study of 45 fetuses, subsequently shown to be normal at birth. Blood samples were obtained by ultrasound-guided cordocentesis.

	SI units (mean ± SD)	Traditional units (mean ± SD)
Glucose	4.3 ± 0.6 mmol/L	7.7 ± 1.1 mg/dL
Cholesterol	1.5 ± 0.3 mmol/L	59 ± 11 mg/dL
Uric acid	179 ± 39 µmol/L	2.8 ± 0.6 mg/dL
Triglycerides	4.5 ± 1.1 mmol/L	40 ± 10 mg/dL
Total bilirubin	26.3 ± 5.8 µmol/L	1.5 ± 0.3 mg/dL
Alkaline phosphatase	260 ± 65 IU/L	
Gamma glutamyl transferase	60 ± 34 IU/L	
Aspartate transaminase	17 ± 6.5 IU/L	
Creatinine	1.8 ± 0.3 µmol/L	0.02 ± 0.003 mg/dL
Calcium	2.3 ± 0.2 mmol/L	9.2 ± 0.8 mg/dL

Figure 72. Glucose, calcium, liver function and renal function tests (mean ± SD) from a cross-sectional study of 78 fetuses of gestational age 20–26 weeks; all fetuses were subsequently shown to be healthy at birth. Blood samples were obtained by ultrasound-guided cordocentesis. *Data source*: ref. 121, with permission.

Renal Function Tests, Liver Function Tests, Glucose

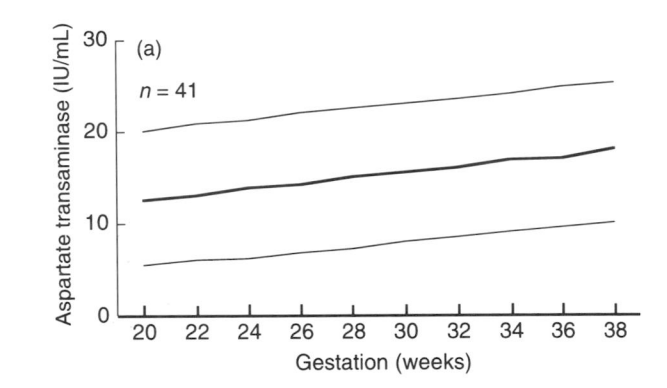 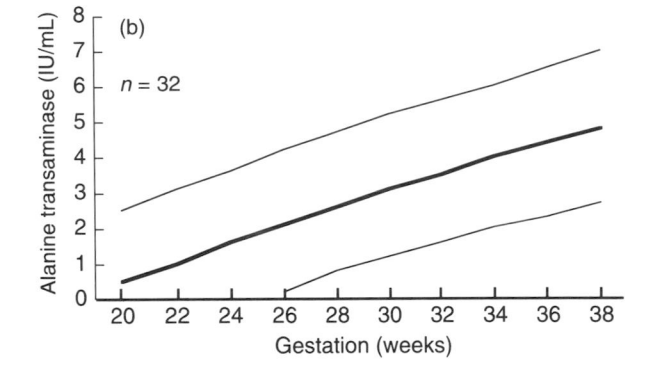

Figure 73. (a) Aspartate transaminase (AST), (b) alanine transaminase (ALT), (c) gamma glutamyl transferase (GGT) and (d) lactate dehydrogenase (LDH) concentrations (regression line and 95% CI) from a cross-sectional study of 80 fetuses referred for assessment of possible intrauterine infection or hemolysis, but subsequently shown to be unaffected. They underwent cordocentesis and blood samples were obtained for liver enzyme assays (the numbers of assays performed for each enzyme are stated on individual graphs). *Data source*: ref. 113, with permission.

Comment: Plasma total protein and albumin concentrations increase significantly with gestational age[120]. Little information is available regarding many of the other biochemical variables: triglyceride levels fall with advancing gestation[121], bilirubin levels rise[122], liver enzyme concentrations (apart from LDH) rise[113]. Fetal concentrations of bilirubin are higher, and those of triglyceride and cholesterol lower, than in maternal serum[121].

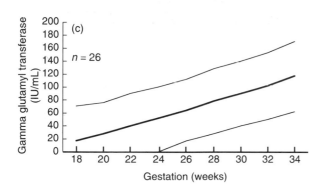

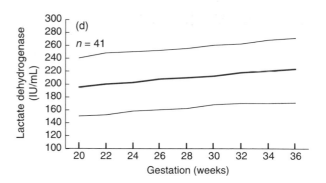

Urinary Biochemistry

(a)	16 weeks	33 weeks
Phosphate (mmol/L)	0.91	0.10
Creatinine (μmol/L)	99.9	172.9
(mean values)		

(b)	Mean value	95% confidence intervals (CI)
Potassium (mmol/L)	3.0	0–6.1
Calcium (mmol/L)	0.21	0.04–1.2
Urea (μmol/L)	7.9	2.6–13.1

◀ **Figure 74**. Urinary electrolytes – (a) phosphate, creatinine, (b) potassium, calcium, urea, (c) sodium (mean and 95% CI where computed) from a study of 26 women between 16 and 33 weeks gestation, with normal amniotic fluid volume and normal fetal anatomy. 17 of the women had pregnancies complicated by Rhesus alloimmunization; in these the fetal bladder was emptied prior to intraperitoneal blood transfusion. The other women had aspiration of the fetal bladder prior to therapeutic termination of pregnancy. *Data source*: ref. 123, with permission.

▼

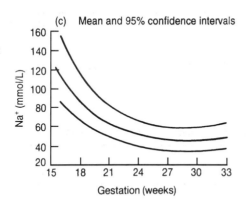

(c) Mean and 95% confidence intervals

Na⁺ (mmol/L) vs Gestation (weeks)

Comment: Fetal urinary biochemistry has previously only been studied indirectly from examination of the amniotic fluid[109]. This direct study found that urinary sodium and phosphate levels decreased significantly with gestational age over the period studied (16–33 weeks); creatinine levels increased. Urinary potassium, calcium and urea did not show gestational changes. The pattern of electrolyte changes suggests parallel maturation of both glomerular and tubular function with advancing gestation.

Blood Gases

Oxygen pressure (Po₂), carbon dioxide pressure (Pco₂), pH and base deficit

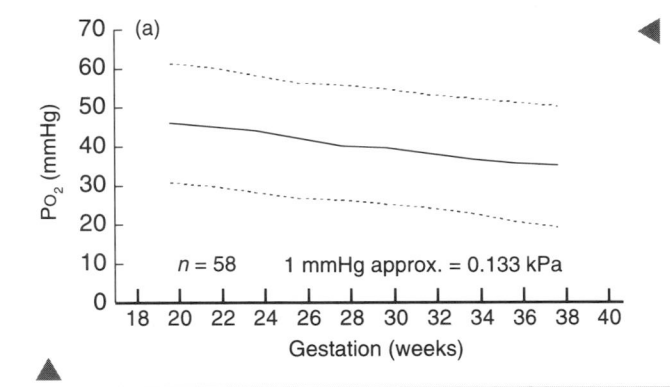

Figure 75. Umbilical venous P_{O_2}, P_{CO_2}, pH and base deficit of the extracellular fluid (2.5th, 50th and 97.5th centiles) from a cross-sectional study of 59 fetuses who had been referred for assessment of possible intrauterine infection or hemolysis, but were found to be unaffected. Subsequently, all were healthy at birth and appropriately grown. *Data source*: ref. 132, with permission.

Comment: Umbilical arterial and venous P_{O_2} and pH decrease, and P_{CO_2} increases with gestational age[124]. Concentrations of lactate do not change with gestation; mean (SD) values are 0.99 (0.32) mmol/L for umbilical vein and 0.92 (0.21) mmol/L for umbilical artery[124]. Intervillous blood has a higher P_{O_2} and lower P_{CO_2}, but similar pH and lactate concentrations as umbilical venous blood[125]. The decrease in P_{O_2} in umbilical venous blood with advancing gestation is offset by increasing fetal hemoglobin concentration, such that blood oxygen content remains constant; mean umbilical venous oxygen content is 6.7 (SD 0.6) mmol/L[125].

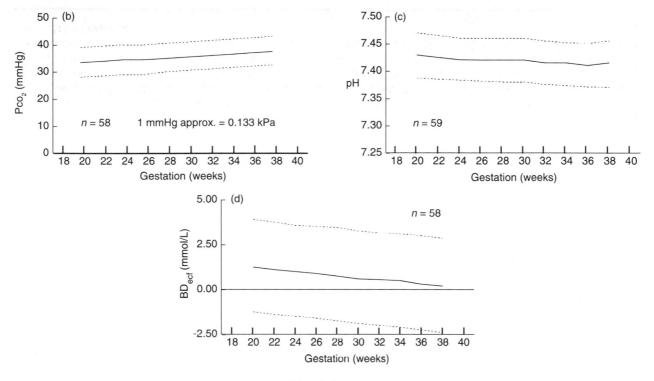

Blood Gases

BIOCHEMISTRY

HEMATOLOGY

Full Blood Count (FBC)

Figure 76. Red cell count (RBC), white cell count (WBC), platelets (PLT), hemoglobin (Hb) and mean cell volume (MCV) from a cross-sectional study of 1233 normal fetuses between 18 and 36 weeks gestation (mean ± SD). These were pregnancies referred for fetal blood sampling for prenatal diagnosis (mostly toxoplasmosis), but the fetuses were normal and subsequently shown to be healthy at birth. Fetal blood samples were taken by ultrasound-guided cordocentesis. *Data source*: ref. 121, with permission.

Gestational age (weeks)	WBC (10^9/L)	PLT (10^9/L)	RBC (10^{12}/L)	Hb (g/dL)	MCV (fL)
18–23 (*n* = 771)	4.41 ± 1.2	241 ± 45	2.87 ± 0.28	11.7 ± 0.8	131.2 ± 7.3
24–29 (*n* = 407)	4.6 ± 1.3	267 ± 49	3.38 ± 0.32	12.8 ± 1.1	119.1 ± 5.6
30–35 (*n* = 55)	5.8 ± 1.6	265 ± 59	3.86 ± 0.43	14.1 ± 1.4	114.3 ± 7

Comment: Fetal red cell count increases with gestation, but white cell count and platelet count do not change[121]. Lymphocytes form the main population of white cells in the fetus; reticulocyte numbers decrease with advancing gestation[121]. Fetal hemoglobin (HbF) decreases with advancing gestation, from over 80% of total hemoglobin in mid-pregnancy to approximately 70% by term[121].

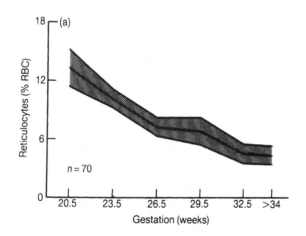

Figure 77. (a) Fetal reticulocyte count (mean and 95% CI) from a cross-sectional study of 81 fetuses referred for prenatal diagnosis for a variety of indications, but subsequently shown to be unaffected. Ultrasound-guided cordocentesis was performed in order to obtain blood samples. *Data source*: ref. 126, with permission.

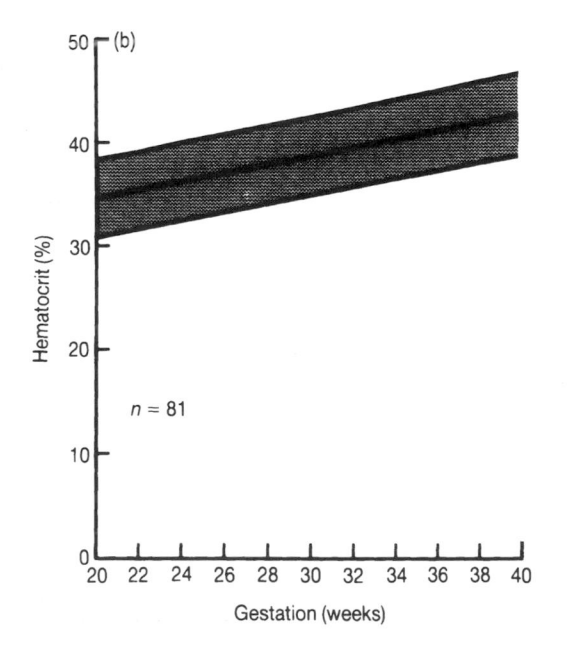

◀ **Figure 77**. (b) Hematocrit (regression line and 95% CI) from a cross-sectional study of 81 fetuses referred for prenatal diagnosis for a variety of indications, but subsequently shown to be unaffected. Ultrasound-guided cordocentesis was performed in order to obtain blood samples. *Data source*: ref. 126, with permission.

Coagulation Factors

Coagulation factors	%	Inhibitors	%
VIIIC	40 ± 12	Fibronectin	40 ± 10
VIIIRAg	60 ± 13	Protein C	11 ± 3
VII	28 ± 5	α_2-Macroglobulin	18 ± 4
IX	9 ± 3	α_1-Antitrypsin	40 ± 4
V	47 ± 10	AT III	30 ± 3
II	12 ± 3	α_2-Antiplasmin	61 ± 6
XII	22 ± 3		
Prekallikrein	19 ± 2		
Fibrin - stabilizing factor	30 ± 5		
Fibrinogen	40 ± 15		
Plasminogen	24 ± 15		

Figure 78. Coagulation factors (percentage of normal adult values; mean ± 1 SD) from a cross-sectional study of 103 fetuses of 19–27 weeks gestational age, subsequently shown to be healthy. Blood samples were obtained by ultrasound-guided cordocentesis. *Data source*: ref. 121, with permission.

Comment: No changes in levels or activity of the various coagulation factors and their inhibitors were observed through the 8 weeks of gestation studied.

Iron Metabolism

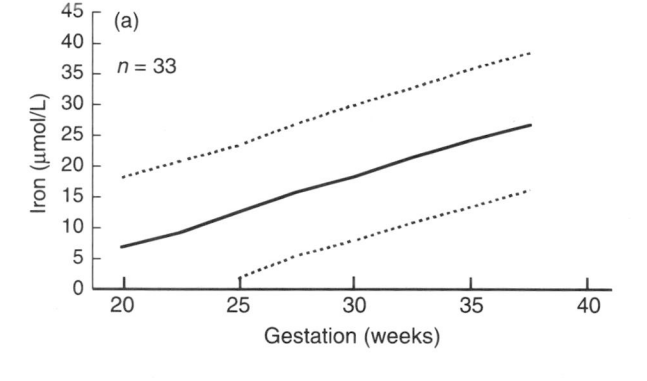

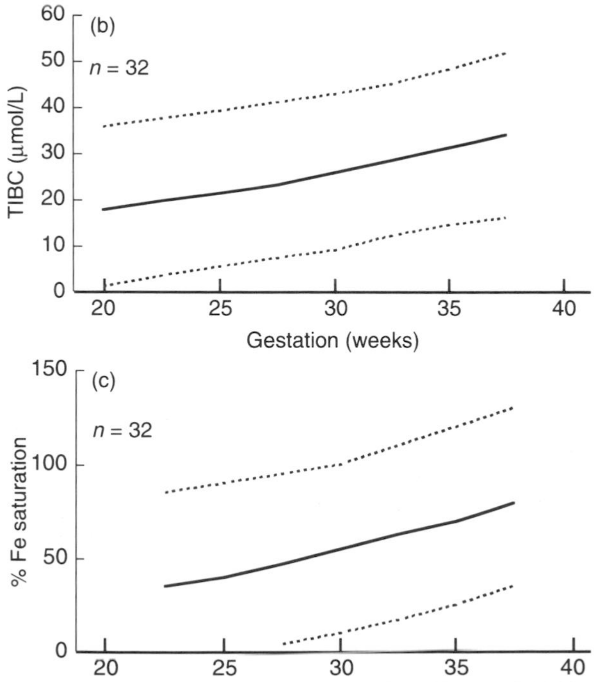

Figure 79. Fetal iron, total iron binding capacity (TIBC) and % iron saturation from a cross-sectional study of 33 fetuses referred for prenatal diagnosis for a variety of indications, but subsequently found to be unaffected. Blood samples were taken by ultrasound-guided cordocentesis. *Data source:* ref. 127, with permission.

Comment: Fetal iron, TIBC and % iron saturation all increase with advancing gestation.

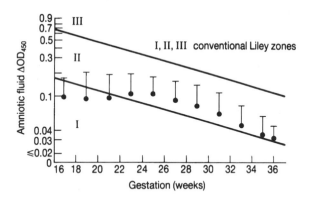

Figure 80. Amniotic fluid bilirubin ΔOD_{450} (mean ± 2 SD) from 475 samples of amniotic fluid obtained from pregnancies between 16 and 36 weeks gestation not complicated by fetal hemolysis. Amniotic fluid samples taken at the time of fetoscopy or by amniocentesis were placed in darkened containers to protect against photodecomposition and centrifuged to remove vernix and cellular debris. The bilirubin concentration was measured spectrophotometrically by the deviation in optical density of the amniotic fluid at a wavelength of 450 nm. *Data source*: ref. 128, with permission.

Comment: The normal range of liquor ΔOD_{450} does not change between the gestational ages of 16 and 25 weeks, but values fall during the third trimester and are widely scattered.

ENDOCRINOLOGY
Thyroid Function

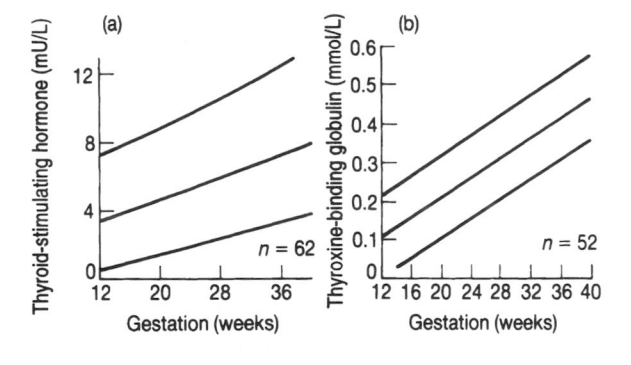

◀ **Figure 81**. Thyroid stimulating hormone (TSH), thyroid binding globulin (TBG), total thyroxine (total T_4), free thyroxine (free T_4), total triiodothyronine (T_3) and free triiodothyronine (T_3) from a study of 62 women who underwent cordocentesis or cardiocentesis for prenatal diagnosis, and whose fetuses were subsequently shown to be normal (mean, 5th, 95th centiles). The cross-hatched area is the lower limit of sensitivity of the assay. *Data source*: ref. 129, with permission.

▼

Comment: No significant associations have been found between fetal and maternal thyroid hormones and TSH concentrations, suggesting that the fetal pituitary-thyroid axis is independent of that of its mother[129]. Fetal TSH levels are always higher than those in the mother. Free and total T_4 levels and those of TBG rise through pregnancy and reach adult levels by 36 weeks gestation; however free and total T_3 levels are always substantially less than adult levels. The increase in fetal blood levels of TSH, thyroid hormones and TBG during pregnancy indicates independent and autonomous maturation of the pituitary, thyroid and liver respectively[129]. There does not appear to be feedback control of pituitary secretion of TSH by circulating thyroid hormones *in utero*.

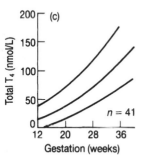
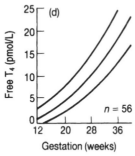
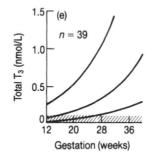
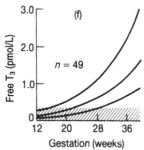

Thyroid Function

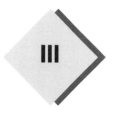

LABOR

Progress of Labor

Figure 82. Mean cervimetric progress from a study of 3217 consecutive women in labor, from which a group of 1306 who had normal labor were identified (i.e. women with a cephalically presenting fetus, who did not have epidural block, receive oxytocic drugs, or require instrumental delivery). The progress of labor was followed by vaginal examination to establish cervical dilatation; the first examination being performed soon after admission to the labor suite. The onset of second stage was confirmed when full cervical dilatation was found at the time of routine examination, or when the patient was beginning to bear down. *Data source*: ref. 130, with permission.

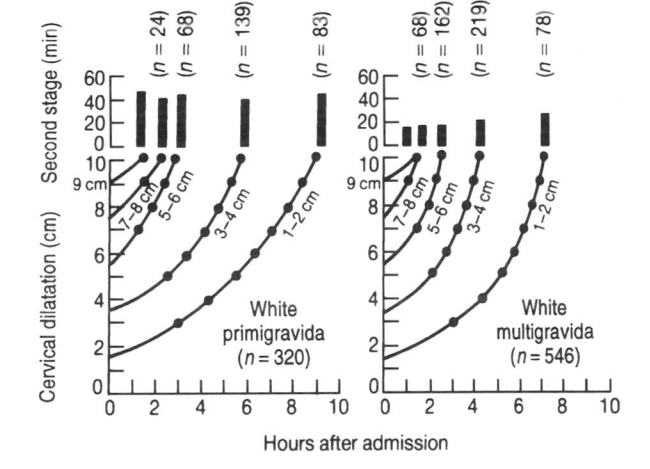

Comment: This study found that mean cervimetric progress from 1 to 7 cm was faster in Caucasian multiparae than primiparae, but thereafter progress in the two groups was similar. No significant differences in the cervimetric progress of labor between women from different racial groups has been found[130]. The mean duration of the second stage of labor is approximately 42 minutes in primiparae and 17 minutes in multiparae[130], although it is recognized that the precise onset of full cervical dilatation is difficult to establish.

Fetal Heart Rate Parameters by Cardiotocography (CTG)

Admission test CTG

- At least two accelerations (>15 beats for >15s) in 20 minutes.
- Baseline heart rate 110–150 bpm.
- Baseline variability 5–25 bpm.
- Absence of decelerations.
- Moderate tachycardia/bradycardia and accelerations.

First stage intrapartum CTG

- At least two accelerations (>15 beats for >15s) in 20 minutes.
- Baseline heart rate 110–150 bpm.
- Baseline variability 5–25 bpm.
- Early decelerations (in late first stage of labor).

Second stage intrapartum CTG

- Normal baseline heart rate, normal baseline variability and no decelerations. Frequent decelerations, both periodic and scattered.
- Baseline heart rate 110–150 bpm and baseline variability 5–25 bpm or >25 bpm, with or without early and/or variable decelerations.

Figure 83. Features of the normal CTG in labor. *Data source*: ref. 117, with permission.

Comment: Decelerations, which are abnormal if identified antepartum (see Figure 69) are often encountered intrapartum. Early decelerations (i.e. synchronous with contractions) are common towards the end of the first stage of labor; during the second stage of labor both early and variable decelerations can be normal findings. Accelerations and normal baseline variability are important features of a healthy CTG.

REFERENCES

1. DAWES MG, GRUDZINKAS JG (1991) Patterns of maternal weight gain in pregnancy. *Br J Obstet Gynaecol* **98**: 195–201.

2. National Academy of Sciences (1990) *Nutrition during Pregnancy.* National Academy Press, Washington DC.

3. ROSSO P (1985) A new chart to monitor weight gain during pregnancy. *Am J Clin Nutr* **41**: 644–652.

4. National Academy of Sciences (1989) *Recommended Dietary Allowances,* 10th edn. National Academy Press, Washington DC.

5. MACGILLIVRAY I, ROSE GA, ROWE B (1969) Blood pressure survey in pregnancy. *Clin Sci* **37**: 395–407.

6. SPATLING L, FALLENSTEIN F, HUCH A, HUCH R, ROOTH G (1992) The variability of cardiopulmonary adaptation to pregnancy at rest and during exercise. *Br J Obstet Gynaecol* **99** (suppl 8).

7. CLAPP JF III (1985) Maternal heart rate in pregnancy. *Am J Obstet Gynecol* **152**: 659–660.

8. CLARK SL, COTTON DB, LEE W, BISHOP C, HILL T, SOUTHWICK J *et al* (1989) Central hemodynamic assessment of normal term pregnancy. *Am J Obstet Gynecol* **161**: 1439–1442.

9. LUCIUS H, GAHLENBECK H, KLEINE H-O, FABEL H, BARTELS H (1970) Respiratory functions, buffer system, and electrolyte concentrations of blood during human pregnancy. *Resp Physiol* **9**: 311–317.

10. GAZIOGLU K, KALTREIDER NL, ROSEN M, YU PN (1970) Pulmonary function during pregnancy in normal women and in patients with cardiopulmonary disease. *Thorax* **25**: 445–450.

11. DE SWIET M (1991) The respiratory system. In: Hytten F, Chamberlain G (eds) *Clinical Physiology in Obstetrics,* 2nd edn, pp. 83–100. Oxford: Blackwell Scientific Publications.

12. CUCKLE HS, WALD NJ and THOMPSON SG (1987) Estimating a woman's risk of having a pregnancy associated with Down's syndrome using her age and serum α-fetoprotein level. *Br J Obstet Gynaecol* **94**: 387–402.

13. FERGUSON-SMITH M (1983) Prenatal chromosome analysis and its impact on the birth incidence of chromosome disorders. *Br Med Bull* **39**: 355–364.

14. ROBERTSON EG, CHEYNE GA (1972) Plasma biochemistry in relation to the oedema of pregnancy. *J Obstet Gynaecol Br Comm* **79**: 769–776.

15. MENDENHALL HW (1970) Serum protein concentrations in pregnancy. *Am J Obstet Gynecol* **106**: 388–399.

16. ADENIYI FA, OLATUNBOSUN DA (1984) Origins and significance of the increased plasma alkaline phosphatase during normal pregnancy and pre-eclampsia. *Br J Obstet Gynaecol* **91**: 857–862.

17. GIRLING J (1995) Personal communication.

18. WALKER FB, HOBLIT DL, CUNNINGHAM FG, COMBES B (1974) Gamma glutamyl transpeptidase in normal pregnancy. *Obstet Gynecol* **43**: 745–749.

19. McNAIR RD, JAYNES RV (1960) Alterations in liver function during normal pregnancy. *Am J Obstet Gynecol* **80**: 500–505.

20. POTTER JM, NESTEL PJ (1979) The hyper-lipidaemia of pregnancy in normal and complicated pregnancies. *Am J Obstet Gynecol* **133**: 165–170.

21. LIND T, GODFREY KA, OTUN H (1984) Changes in serum uric acid concentrations during normal pregnancy. *Br J Obstet Gynaecol* **91**: 128–132.

22. NEWMAN RL (1957) Serum electrolytes in pregnancy, parturition, and puerperium. *Obstet Gynecol* **10**: 51–55.

23. KUHLBACK B, WIDHOLM O (1966) Plasma creatinine in normal pregnancy. *Scand J Clin Lab Invest* **18**: 654–656.

24. DAVISON J (1989) Renal disease. In: de Swiet M (ed.) *Medical Disorders in Obstetric Practice,* 2nd edn, pp. 306–407. Oxford: Blackwell Scientific Publications.

25. DAVISON JM, NOBLE MCB (1981) Serial changes in 24 hour creatinine clearance during normal menstrual cycles and the first trimester of pregnancy. *Br J Obstet Gynaecol* **88**: 10–17.

26. DAVISON JM, DUNLOP W, EZIMOKHAI M (1980) 24-hour creatinine clearance during the third trimester of normal pregnancy. *Br J Obstet Gynaecol* **87**: 106–109.

27. DAVISON JM, DUNLOP W (1980) Renal haemo-dynamics and tubular function in normal human pregnancy. *Kidney Int* **18**: 152–161.

28. HYTTEN FE, CHEYNE GA (1972) The amino-aciduria of pregnancy. *J Obstet Gynaecol Br Comm* **79**: 424–432.

29. LOPEZ-ESPINOLA I, DHAR H, HUMPHREYS S, REDMAN CWG (1986) Urinary albumin excretion in pregnancy. *Br J Obstet Gynaecol* **93**: 176–181.

30. LIND T, BILLEWICZ WZ, BROWN G (1973) A serial study of changes occuring in the oral glucose tolerance test during pregnancy. *J Obstet Gynaecol Br Comm* **80**: 1033–1039.

31. HATEM M, ANTHONY F, HOGSTON P, ROWE DJF, DENNIS KJ (1988) Reference values for 75 g oral glucose tolerance test in pregnancy. *Br Med J* **296**: 676–678.

32. O'SULLIVAN JB, MAHAN CM (1964) Criteria for the oral glucose tolerance test in pregnancy. *Diabetes* **13**: 278–285.

33. ROBERTS AB, BAKER JR (1986) Serum fructosamine: a screening test for diabetes in pregnancy. *Am J Obstet Gynecol* **154**: 1027–1030.

34. FEIGE A, NOSSNER U (1985) Das Verhalten des glykosylierten Haemoglobins (Hb-A1) in normaler und pathologischer Schwangerschaft. *Z Geburtshilfe Perinatol* **189**: 13–16.

35. YLINEN K, HEKALIR R, TERAMO K (1981) Haemoglobin A_{1c} during pregnancy of insulin-dependent diabetic and healthy control. *J Obstet Gynaecol* **1**: 223–228.

36. TAYLOR DJ, LIND T (1979) Red cell mass during and after normal pregnancy. *Br J Obstet Gynaecol* **86**: 364–370.

37. EFRATI P, PRESENTEY B, MARGALITH M, ROZENSZAJN L (1964) Leukocytes of normal pregnant women. *Obstet Gynecol* **23**: 429–432.

38. KUVIN SF, BRECHER G (1962) Differential neutrophil counts in pregnancy. *N Engl J Med* **266**: 877–878.

39. FAY RA, HUGHES AO, FARRON NT (1983) Platelets in pregnancy: hyperdestruction in pregnancy. *Obstet Gynecol* **61**: 238–240.

platelet count in pregnancy. *J Clin Pathol* **30**: 68–69.

41. FENTON V, CAVILL I, FISHER J (1977) Iron stores in pregnancy. *Br J Haematol* **37**: 145–149.

42. EK J, MAGNUS M (1981) Plasma and red blood cell folate during normal pregnancies. *Acta Obstet Gynecol Scand* **60**: 247–251.

43. CHANARIN I, ROTHMAN D, WARD A, PERRY J (1968) Folate status and requirement in pregnancy. *Br Med J* **2**: 390–394.

44. LETSKY E (1991) The haematological system. In: Hytten F, Chamberlain G (eds) *Clinical Physiology in Obstetrics,* 2nd edn, pp. 39–82. Oxford: Blackwell Scientific Publications.

45. TEMPERLEY IJ, MEEHAN MJM, GATENBY PBB (1968) Serum vitamin B12 levels in pregnant women. *J Obstet Gynaecol Br Comm* **75**: 511–516.

46. STIRLING Y, WOOLF L, NORTH WRS, SEGHATCHIAN MJ, MEADE TW (1984) Haemostasis in normal pregnancy. *Thromb Haemost* **52**: 176–182.

47. WARWICK R, HUTTON HA, GOFF L, LETSKY E, HEARD M (1989) Changes in protein C and free protein S during pregnancy and following hysterectomy. *J R Soc Med* **82**:591–594.

48. BONNAR J, MCNICOL GP, DOUGLAS AS (1969) Fibrinolytic enzyme system and pregnancy. *Br Med J* **iii**: 387–389.

49. GALLERY ED, RAFTOS J, GYORY AZ, WELLS JV (1981) A prospective study of serum complement (C3 and C4) levels during normal human pregnancy: effect of the development of pregnancy-associated hypertension. *Aust NZ J Med* **11**: 243–245.

50. SCHENA FP, MANNO C, SELVAGGI L, LOVERRO G, BETTOCCHI S, BONOMO L (1982) Behaviour of immune complexes and the complement system in normal pregnancy and pre-eclampsia. *J Clin Lab Immunol* **7**: 21–26.

51. JENKINS JS, POWELL RJ (1987) C3 degradation products (C3d) in normal pregnancy. *J Clin Pathol* **40**: 1362–1363.

52. HYTTEN FE, LIND T (1973) Volume and composition of the blood. In: *Diagnostic Indices in Pregnancy*, pp. 36–54. Basle, Switzerland: Documenta Geigy.

53. HARADA A, HERSHMAN JM, REED AW *et al.* (1979) Comparison of thyroid stimulators and thyroid hormone concentrations in the sera of pregnant women. *J Clin Endocrinol Metab* **48**: 793–797.

54. MAN EB, REID WA, HELLEGERS AE, JONES WS (1969) Thyroid function in human pregnancy. *Am J Obstet Gynecol* **103**: 338–347.

55. PARKER JH (1985) Amerlex free triiodothyronine and free thyroxine levels in normal pregnancy. *Br J Obstet Gynaecol* **92**: 1234–1238.

56. OSATHANONDH R, TULCHINSKY D, CHOPRA IJ (1976) Total and free thyroxine and triiodothyronine in normal and complicated pregnancy. *J Clin Endocrinol Metab* **42**: 98–102.

57. NATRAJAN PG, McGARRIGLE HHG, LAWRENCE DM, LACHELIN GCL (1982) Plasma noradrenaline and adrenaline levels in normal pregnancy and in pregnancy-induced hypertension. *Br J Obstet Gynaecol* **89**: 1041–1045.

58. RUBIN PC, BUTTERS L, McCABE R, REID JL (1986) Plasma catecholamines in pregnancy-induced hypertension. *Clin Sci* **71**: 111–115.

59. BEILIN LJ, DEACON J, MICHAEL CA *et al* (1983) Diurnal rhythms of blood pressure, plasma renin activity, angiotensin II and catecholamines in normotensive and hypertensive pregnancies. *Clin Exp Hypertension – Hypertension in Pregnancy* **B2** (2): 271–293.

60. CARR BR, PARKER CR, MADDEN JD, MACDONALD PC, PORTER JC (1981) Maternal plasma adrenocorticotrophin and cortisol relationships throughout human pregnancy. *Am J Obstet Gynecol* **139**: 416–422.

61. NOLTEN WE, LINDHEIMER MD, RUECKERT PA, OPARIL S, EHRLICH EN (1980) Diurnal patterns and regulation of cortisol secretion in pregnancy. *J Clin Endocrinol Metab* **51**: 466–472.

62. REES LH, BURKE CW, CHARD T, EVANS SW, LETCHWORTH AT (1975) Possible placental origin of ACTH in normal human pregnancy. *Nature* **254**: 620–622.

63. DOE RP, FERNANDEZ R, SEAL US (1964) Measurement of corticosteroid-binding globulin in man. *J Clin Endocrinol* **24**: 1029–1039.

64. MIGEON CJ, KENNY FM, TAYLOR FH (1968)

Cortisol production rate VIII. Pregnancy. *J Clin Endocrinol* **28**: 661–666.

65. PEARSON MURPHY BE, OKOUNEFF LM, KLEIN GP, NGO SH (1981) Lack of specificity of cortisol determinations in human urine. *J Clin Endocrinol Metab* **53**: 91–99.

66. NOLTEN WE, LINDHEIMER MD, OPARIL S, EHRLICH EN (1978) Desoxycorticosterone in normal pregnancy. I. Sequential studies of the secretory patterns of desoxycorticosterone, aldosterone, and cortisol. *Am J Obstet Gynecol* **132**: 414–420.

67. GARNER PR (1995) Pituitary and adrenal disorders. In: Burrow GN, Ferris TF (eds) *Medical Complications during Pregnancy,* 4th edn, pp. 188–209. Philadelphia: WB Saunders.

68. BISWAS S, RODEK CH (1976) Plasma prolactin levels during pregnancy. *Br J Obstet Gynaecol* **83**: 683–687.

69. BOYER RM, FINKELSTEIN JW, KAPEN S, HELLMAN L (1975) Twenty-four hour prolactin (Prl) secretory patterns during pregnancy. *J Clin Endocrinol Metab* **40**: 1117–1120.

70. RIGG LA, YEN SSC (1977) Multiphasic prolactin secretion during parturition in human subjects. *Am J Obstet Gynecol* **128**: 215–218.

71. JACOBS HS (1991) The hypothalamus and pituitary gland. In: Hytten F, Chamberlain G (eds) *Clinical Physiology in Obstetrics,* 2nd edn, pp. 345–356. Oxford: Blackwell Scientific Publications.

72. PITKIN RM, REYNOLDS WA, WILLIAMS GA, HARGIS GK (1979) Calcium metabolism in normal pregnancy: a longitudinal study. *Am J Obstet Gynecol* **133**: 781–787.

73. SEKI K, MAKIMURA N, MITSUI C, HIRATA J, NAGATA I (1991) Calcium-regulating hormones and osteocalcin levels during pregnancy: a longitudinal study. *Am J Obstet Gynecol* **164**: 1248–1252.

74. SEPPALA M, RUOSLAHTI E (1972) Radioimmunoassay of maternal alpha fetoprotein during pregnancy and delivery. *Am J Obstet Gynecol* **112**: 208–212.

75. HADDOW JE, PALOMAKI GE (1992) Maternal protein enzyme analyses. In: Reece EA, Hobbins JC, Mahoney MJ, Petrie RH (eds) *Medicine of the Fetus and Mother,* pp. 653–667. Philadelphia: JB Lippincott Company.

76. BATZER FR, SCHLAFF S, GOLDFARB AF, CORSON SL (1981) Serial ß-subunit human chorionic gonadotrophin doubling time as a prognosticator of pregnancy outcome in an infertile population. *Fertil Steril* **35**: 307–311.

77. BRODY S, CARLSTROM G (1965) Human chorionic gonadotrophin pattern in serum and its relation to the sex of the fetus. *J Clin Endocrinol* **25**: 792–797.

78. JOSIMOVICH JB, KOSOR B, BOCCELLA L, MINTZ DH, HUTCHINSON DL (1970) Placental lactogen in maternal serum as an index of fetal health. *Obstet Gynecol* **36**: 244–250.

79. BECK P, PARKER ML, DAUGHADAY WH (1965) Radioimmunologic measurement of human placental lactogen in plasma by a double antibody method during normal and diabetic pregnancies. *J Clin Endocrinol* **25**: 1457–1462.

80. MATHUR RS, LEAMING AB, WILLIAMSON HO (1972) A simplified method for estimation of estriol in pregnancy plasma. *Am J Obstet Gynecol* **113**: 1120–1129.

81. MILLS MS (1992) Ultrasonography of early embryonic growth and fetal development. MD Thesis, University of Bristol.

82. ROBINSON HP, FLEMING JEE (1975) A critical evaluation of sonar 'crown-rump length' measurements. *Br J Obstet Gynaecol* **82**: 702–710.

83. PEDERSEN JF (1982) Fetal crown-rump length measurement by ultrasound in normal pregnancy. *Br J Obstet Gynaecol* **89**: 926–930.

84. PARKER AJ, DAVIES P, NEWTON JR (1982) Assessment of gestational age of the Asian fetus by the sonar measurement of crown-rump length and biparietal diameter. *Br J Obstet Gynaecol* **89**: 836–838.

85. ERIKSON PS, SECHER NJ, WEIS-BENTZON M (1985) Normal growth of the fetal biparietal diameter and the abdominal diameter in a longitudinal study. *Acta Obstet Gynecol Scand* **64**: 65–70.

86. CHITTY LS, ALTMAN DG (1993) Charts of fetal size. In: Dewbury K, Meire H, Cosgrove D (eds) *Ultrasound in Obstetrics and Gynaecology*, pp. 513–595. Edinburgh: Churchill Livingstone.

87. HADLOCK FP, DETER RL, HARRIST RB, PARK SK (1982) Fetal head circumference: relation to menstrual age. *Am J Roentgenol* **138**: 647–653.

88. DETER RL, HARRIST RB, HADLOCK FP, POINDEXTER AN (1982) Longitudinal studies of fetal growth with the use of dynamic image ultrasonography. *Am J Obstet Gynecol* **143**: 545–554.

89. HADLOCK FP, DETER RL, HARRIST RB, PARK SK (1982) Fetal abdominal circumference as a predictor of menstrual age. *Am J Roentgenol* **139**: 367–370.

90. DETER RL, HARRIST RB, HADLOCK FP, CARPENTER RJ (1982) Fetal head and abdominal circumferences: II A critical re-evaluation of the relationship to menstrual age. *J Clin Ultrasound* **10**: 365–372.

91. WARDA AH, DETER RL, ROSSAVIK IK, CARPENTER RJ, HADLOCK FP (1985) Fetal femur length: a critical reevaluation of the relationship to menstrual age. *Obstet Gynecol* **66**: 69–75.

92. SHALEV E, FELDMAN E, WEINER E, ZUCKERMAN H (1985) Assessment of gestational age by ultrasonic measurement of the femur length. *Acta Obstet Gynecol Scand* **64**: 71–74.

93. MERZ E, KIM-KERN M-S, PEHL S (1987) Ultrasonic mensuration of fetal limb bones in the second and third trimesters. *J Clin Ultrasound* **15**: 175–183.

94. JEANTY P (1991) Fetal biometry. In: Fleischer AC, Romero R, Manning FA, Jeanty P, James AE (eds) *The Principles and Practice of Ultrasonography in Obstetrics and Gynecology,* 4th edn, pp. 93–108. Norwalk, Connecticut: Appleton and Lange.

95. ROMERO R, ATHANASSIADIS AP, SIRTORI M, INATI M (1991) Fetal skeletal anomalies. In: Fleischer AC, Romero R, Manning FA, Jeanty P, James AE (eds) *The Principles and Practice of Ultrasonography in Obstetrics and Gynecology,* 4th edn, pp. 277–306. Norwalk, Connecticut: Appleton and Lange.

96. GRANNUM P, BRACKEN M, SILVERMAN R, HOBBINS JC (1980) Assessment of fetal kidney size in normal gestation by comparison of ratio of kidney circumference to abdominal circumference. *Am J Obstet Gynecol* **136**: 249–254.

97. MAYDEN KL, TORTORA M, BERKOWITZ RL, BRACKEN M, HOBBINS JC (1982) Orbital diameters: a new parameter for prenatal diagnosis and dating. *Am J Obstet Gynecol* **144**: 289–297.

REFERENCES

98. CAMPBELL S. Personal communication. Data from the Ultrasound Department at King's College Hospital, London, UK.

99. GOLDSTEIN I, REECE EA, PILU G, BOVICELLI L, HOBBINS JC (1987) Cerebellar measurements with ultrasonography in the evaluation of fetal growth and development. *Am J Obstet Gynecol* **156**: 1065–1069.

100. THOMPSON AM, BILLEWICZ WZ, HYTTEN FE (1968) The assessment of fetal growth. *J Obstet Gynaecol Br Comm* **75**: 903–916.

101. WILLIAMS RL, CREASY RK, CUNNINGHAM GC, HAWES WE, NORRIS FD, TASHIRO M (1982) Fetal growth and perinatal viability in California. *Obstet Gynecol* **59**: 624–632.

102. CAMPBELL S, WILKIN D (1975) Ultrasonic measurement of fetal abdomen circumference in the estimation of fetal weight. *Br J Obstet Gynaecol* **82**: 689–697.

103. SHEPARD MJ, RICHARDS VA, BERKOWITZ RL, WARSOF SL, HOBBINS JC (1982) An evaluation of two equations for predicting fetal weight by ultrasound. *Am J Obstet Gynecol* **142**: 47–54.

104. HADLOCK FP, HARRIST RB, CARPENTER RJ, DETER RL, PARK SK (1984) Sonographic estimation of fetal weight. *Radiology* **150**: 535–540.

105. BRACE RA, WOLF EJ (1989) Normal amniotic fluid volume changes throughout pregnancy. *Am J Obstet Gynecol* **161**: 382–388.

106. MOORE TR, CAYLE JE (1990) The amniotic fluid index in normal human pregnancy. *Am J Obstet Gynecol* **162**: 1168–1173.

107. FISK NM, RONDEROS-DUMIT D, TANNIRANDORN Y, NICOLINI U, TALBERT D (1992) Normal amniotic pressure throughout gestation. *Br J Obstet Gynaecol* **99**: 18–22.

108. GILBERT WM, MOORE TR, BRACE RA (1991) Amniotic fluid volume dynamics. *Fetal Med Rev* **3**: 89–104.

109. LIND T, PARKIN FM, CHEYNE GA (1969) Biochemical and cytological changes in liquor amnii with advancing gestation. *J Obstet Gynaecol Br Comm* **76**: 673–683.

110. RIZZO G, CAPPONI A, ARDUINI D, ROMANINI C (1994) Ductus venosus velocity waveforms in appropriate and small for gestational age fetuses. *Early Hum Dev* **39**: 15–26.

111. ERSKINE RLA, RITCHIE JWK (1985) Umbilical artery blood flow characteristics in normal and growth-retarded fetuses. *Br J Obstet Gynaecol* **92**: 605–610.

112. RIZZO G, ARDUINI D (1991) Fetal cardiac function in intrauterine growth retardation. *Am J Obstet Gynecol* **165**: 876–882.

113. WEINER CP, SIPES SL, WENSTROM K (1992) The effect of fetal age upon normal fetal laboratory values and venous pressure. *Obstet Gynecol* **79**: 713–718.

114. WEINER CP, HEILSKOV J, PELZER G, GRANT S, WENSTROM K, WILLIAMSON RA (1989) Normal values for human umbilical venous and amniotic fluid pressures and their alteration by fetal disease. *Am J Obstet Gynecol* **161**: 714–717.

115. WEINER CP (1995) Intrauterine pressure: amniotic and fetal circulation. In: Ludomirski A, Nicolini U, Bhutani UK (eds) *Therapeutic and Diagnostic Interventions in Early Life,* Chapter 4. New York: Futura Publishing Co Inc.

116. SADOVSKY G, NICOLAIDES KH (1989) Reference ranges for fetal heart rate patterns in normoxaemic nonanaemic fetuses. *Fetal Ther* **4**: 61–68.

117. ARULKUMARAN S, INGEMARSSON I, MONTAN S, GIBB DMF, PAUL R, SCHIFRIN B, SPENCER JAD, STEER PJ (1992) *Guidelines for Interpretation of Antepartum and Intrapartum Cardiotocography.* Bracknell, Berks: Hewlett Packard.

118. MANNING FA, PLATT LD, SIPOS L (1980) Antepartum fetal evaluation: Development of a fetal biophysical profile. *Am J Obstet Gynecol* **136**: 787–795.

119. MANNING FA, BASKETT TF, MORRISON I, LANGE I (1981) Fetal biophysical profile scoring: A prospective study in 1184 high-risk patients. *Am J Obstet Gynecol* **140**: 289–294.

120. TAKAGI K, TANAKA H, NISHIJIMA S, MASOAKA N, MIYAKE Y, SAKATA H, SATOH K (1989) Fetal blood values by percutaneous umbilical blood sampling. *Fetal Ther* **4**: 152–160.

121. FORESTIER F (1987) Some aspects of fetal biology. *Fetal Ther* **2**: 181–187.

122. WEINER CP (1992) Human fetal bilirubin levels and fetal hemolytic disease. *Am J Obstet Gynecol* **166**: 1449–1454.

123. NICOLINI U, FISK NM, RODECK CH, BEACHAM J (1992) Fetal urine biochemistry: an index of renal maturation and dysfunction. *Br J Obstet Gynaecol* **99**: 46–50.

124. NICOLAIDES KH, ECONOMIDES DL, SOOTHILL PW (1989) Blood gases, pH, and lactate in appropriate- and small-for-gestational-age fetuses. *Am J Obstet Gynecol* **161**: 996–1001.

125. SOOTHILL PW, NICOLAIDES KH, RODECK CH, CAMPBELL S (1986) Effect of gestational age on fetal and intervillous blood gas and acid-base values in human pregnancy. *Fetal Ther* **1**: 168–175.

126. WEINER CP, WILLIAMSON RA, WENSTROM KD, SIPES SL, GRANT SS, WIDNESS JA (1991) Management of fetal hemolytic disease by cordocentesis. I. Prediction of fetal anemia. *Am J Obstet Gynecol* **165**: 546–553.

127. WEINER CP (1995) Unpublished data.

128. NICOLAIDES KH, RODECK CH, MIBASHAN RS, KEMP JR (1986) Have Liley charts outlived their usefulness? *Am J Obstet Gynecol* **155**: 90–94.

129. THORPE-BEESTON JG, NICOLAIDES KH, FELTON CV, BUTLER J, MCGREGOR AM (1991) Maturation of the secretion of thyroid hormone and thyroid stimulating hormone in the fetus. *N Engl J Med* **324**: 532–536.

130. DUIGNAN NM, STUDD JWW, HUGHES AO (1975) Characteristics of normal labour in different racial groups. *Br J Obstet Gynaecol* **82**: 593–601.

131. DICKINSON JE, PALMER SM (1990) Gestational diabetes: pathophysiology and diagnosis. *Seminars in Perinatology* **14**: 2–11.

132. HUCH A, HUCH R, ROOTH G (1994) Guidelines for blood sampling and measurement of pH and blood gas values in obstetrics. *Eur J Obstet Gynaecol Reprod Biol* **54**: 165–175.

INDEX